BLUEPRINTS
DERMATOLOGY

Blueprints **for your pocket!**

In an effort to answer a need for high yield review books for the elective rotations, Blackwell Publishing now brings you Blueprints in pocket size.

These new Blueprints provide the essential content needed during the shorter rotations. They will also provide the basic content needed for USMLE Steps 2 and 3. If you want basic content but were unable to fit in the rotation, these new pocket-sized Blueprints are just what you need.

Each book will focus on the high yield essential content for the most commonly encountered problems of the specialty. Each book features these special appendices:

- Career and residency opportunities
- Commonly prescribed medications
- Self-test Q&A section

Ask for these at your medical bookstore or check them out online at www.blackwellmedstudent.com

Blueprints Dermatology
Blueprints Urology
Blueprints Pediatric Infectious Diseases
Blueprints Ophthalmology
Blueprints Plastic Surgery
Blueprints Orthopedics
Blueprints Hematology and Oncology
Blueprints Anesthesiology
Blueprints Infectious Diseases

BLUEPRINTS
DERMATOLOGY

Rebecca B. Campen, M.D., J.D.
Assistant Professor of Dermatology
Harvard Medical School
Boston, Massachusetts

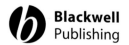
Blackwell
Publishing

© 2004 by Rebecca B. Campen, MD

Blackwell Publishing, Inc., 350 Main Street, Malden, Massachusetts
02148-5018, USA
Blackwell Publishing Ltd, 9600 Garsington Road, Oxford OX4 2DQ, UK
Blackwell Publishing Asia Pty Ltd, 550 Swanston Street, Carlton, Victoria
3053, Australia

04 05 06 07 5 4 3 2 1

ISBN: 1-4051-0441-4

Library of Congress Cataloging-in-Publication Data

Campen, Rebecca B.
  Blueprints dermatology/Rebecca B. Campen.
      p.;   cm. — (Blueprints)
  Includes index.
  ISBN 1-4051-0441-4 (pbk.)
  1. Dermatology—Handbooks, manuals, etc. 2. Dermatology—Outlines,
syllabi, etc. 3. Skin—Diseases—Handbooks, manuals, etc. 4. Skin—
Diseases–Outlines, syllabi, etc.
  [DNLM: 1. Skin Diseases—Handbooks. 2. Skin Diseases—Outlines.
3. Dermatologic Agents—Handbooks. 4. Dermatologic Agents—Outlines.
5. Skin Care—Handbooks. 6. Skin Care—Outlines. WR 18.2 C186 2004]
I. Title. II. Series.

  RL74.C346 2004
  616.5—dc22

                                                    2004003923

A catalogue record for this title is available from the British Library

Acquisitions: Beverly Copland
Development: Selene Steneck
Production: Debra Murphy
Cover design: Hannus Design Associates
Interior design: Mary McKeon
Illustrations: Electronic Illustrators Group
Typesetter: International Typesetting and Composition in Ft.Lauderdale, FL
Printed and bound by Walsworth Publishing Co. in Marceline, MO

For further information on Blackwell Publishing, visit our website:
www.blackwellmedstudent.com

Notice: The indications and dosages of all drugs in this book have been recommended in the medical literature and conform to the practices of the general community. The medications described do not necessarily have specific
approval by the Food and Drug Administration for use in the diseases and
dosages for which they are recommended. The package insert for each drug
should be consulted for use and dosage as approved by the FDA. Because
standards for usage change, it is advisable to keep abreast of revised recom-
mendations, particularly those concerning new drugs.

This book is dedicated to my husband, Tom.

Contents

Reviewers

Tatiana M. Grzeszkiewicz, MD, PhD
Intern, Internal Medicine
UIC-Christ Internal Medicine
Chicago, Illinois

Amanda Kimbrough
Class of 2004
The University of Texas Health Science Center at San Antonio
San Antonio, Texas

Rachel Shemtov
Class of 2004
Yale Medical School
New Haven, Connecticut

Rashmi P. Lodha, MD
PGY-1
Jackson Memorial Hospital
Miami, Florida

Nkiruka Ohameje
Class of 2004
Drexel University College of Medicine
Philadelphia, Pennsylvania

Arne Olsen
Class of 2004
Medical College of Wisconsin
Milwaukee, Wisconsin

Rebecca Smith
Class of 2005
MD/MBA Program
University of California–Irvine
Irvine, California

Preface

Blueprints have become the standard for medical students to use during their clerkship rotations and sub-internships and as a review book before taking the USMLE Steps 2 and 3.

Blueprints initially were only available for the five main specialties: medicine, pediatrics, obstetrics and gynecology, surgery, and psychiatry. Students found these books so valuable that they asked for Blueprints in other topics and so family medicine, emergency medicine, neurology, cardiology and radiology were added.

In an effort to answer a need for high yield review books for the elective rotations, Blackwell Publishing now brings you Blueprints in pocket size. These books are developed to provide students in the shorter, elective rotations—often taken in 4th year—with the same high yield, essential contents of the larger Blueprints books. These new pocket-sized Blueprints will be invaluable for those students who need to know the essentials of a clinical area but were unable to take the rotation. Students in physician assistant, nurse practitioner, and osteopath programs will find these books meet their needs for the clinical specialties.

Feedback from student reviewers gives high praise for this addition to the Blueprints brand. Each of these new books was developed to be read in a short time period and to address the basics needed during a particular clinical rotation. Please see the Series Page for a list of the books that will soon be in your bookstore.

Acknowledgments

I am grateful to Dr. Howard Baden for allowing me to use his outstanding library of clinical photographs for the book and to Dr. Arthur Sober for his very thorough review of the manuscript. I am grateful to my husband, Dr. Thomas Campen, for his encouragement to write this book, and to my three children, Christy Bedingfield, Esq., Dr. Marvin Bradford Bedingfield, and Herbert Marvin Bedingfield, Esq., who continue to encourage and inspire my writing. I am also grateful to my mother and father, Mr. and Mrs. Fred Birchmore, for their encouragement, wisdom, and confidence that continues to inspire me, and to my sister, Dr. Melinda Musick, also a dermatologist, for her wise input into this book. I would also like to thank Beverly Copland, Selene Steneck, and Debra Murphy at Blackwell Publishing, Inc. for their tireless editing and advice, as well as those others who have reviewed, made suggestions, and encouraged the writing of this book. Their efforts have made the book possible.

—Rebecca B. Campen, M.D., J.D.

Abbreviations

AIDS	acquired immunodeficiency syndrome
ANA	antinuclear antibody
ANCA	autoantibodies against neutrophil cytoplasmic antigens
bid	twice a day
CDC	Centers for Disease Control and Prevention
CTCL	cutaneous T-cell lymphoma
DHEAS	dehydroepiandrosterone sulfate
ER	emergency room
FDA	U.S. Food and Drug Administration
FSH	follicle-stimulating hormone
HHV-8	human herpesvirus type 8
HIV	human immunodeficiency virus
HPV	human papillomavirus
IgE	immunoglobulin E
IgG	immunoglobulin G
IgM	immunoglobulin M
KOH	potassium hydroxide
LH	luteinizing hormone
MRI	magnetic resonance imaging
NaCl	sodium chloride
NF1	neurofibromatosis type 1
NF2	neurofibromatosis type 2
po	by mouth
PUVA	psoralens plus UVA
qam	in the morning
qd	once a day
qid	four times a day
qpm	at night
RPR	rapid plasma reagin (test)
SPF	sun protective factor
TEN	toxic epidermal necrolyis
tid	three times a day
UVA	ultraviolet light in the range of 320 to 400 nm wavelength
UVB	ultraviolet light in the range of 280 to 320 nm wavelength

1

Evaluation of a Dermatologic Patient

Examining the Patient

When examining a patient with a dermatologic problem, first note the appearance, location, and distribution of the lesion(s). Determine the primary lesion, secondary changes, distribution, and configuration (Table 1-1). Feel the lesion. Is it superficial or deep, rough or smooth, thin or thick? Is it moveable or fixed? Is it soft, compressible, or hard? Does it blanch (turn from pink to white) when pressed?

Ask the patient about the problem: when the lesion first appeared, how it looked initially, how it has changed, and if it itches, hurts, stings, or burns. Ask if there are any systemic symptoms such as sore throat, runny nose, cough. Ask how the problem has been treated and whether the treatment has helped. If the problem is a rash, ask if it is worse during the day or night, weekdays or weekends, or during certain seasons. Ask if any other family members have this problem. Ask what kind of skin products the patient uses and whether the patient has problems with dry skin.

Diagnostic Tools

Microscopic examination is often performed to assess the skin for fungi, scabies, viral-induced giant cells, bacteria, or yeast. Scrape skin onto a glass slide using a No. 15 blade. If fungal infection is suspected, add a drop of potassium hydroxide (KOH), heat gently under a flame, and examine under the microscope. Look for fungal hyphae and distinguish from cell walls in the sample. If scabies is suspected, add mineral oil instead of KOH to skin scrapings and do not warm the slide. Scrape deeper than for a fungal scraping to see the scabies mite in the stratum corneum. To detect giant cells (intracytoplasmic edema in keratinocytes) found in varicella zoster, or multinucleated ghost cells (nuclei of keratinocytes that have dissolved) in herpesvirus infections, scrape skin from the base of a vesicle (Tzanck preparation) and stain with Wright-Giemsa. Gram stain of exudate from a lesion can be useful in detecting bacterial or yeast infections (Box 1-1).

A skin culture is helpful when viral, bacterial, or fungal infection is suspected. Use sterile swabs and appropriate medium (check with the laboratory) for the particular type of culture. If a

■ TABLE 1-1 Describing a Skin Lesion

Primary Lesions

Macule	Flat, circumscribed lesion differing in color or appearance from the surrounding skin
Papule	Elevated lesion usually <0.5 cm in diameter
Pustule	Raised lesion with purulent exudate
Patch	Area of skin differing from surrounding skin ; usually >1 cm in diameter
Plaque	Broad, flat, elevated lesions usually >1 cm in diameter
Nodule	Round or dome-shaped, solid lesion >1 cm in diameter
Tumor	Solid lesion similar to nodule but >2 cm in diameter
Vesicle	Elevated lesion containing fluid, usually <1 cm in diameter; tense or flaccid
Bulla	Elevated lesion containing fluid, usually >1 cm in diameter; tense or flaccid
Cyst	Spherical or oval nodule containing fluid or semi-solid material
Rash	General term indicating change in epidermis, may have many different appearances
Wheal	Pale pink or red, elevated plaque or papule disappearing within hours (characteristic of hives)
Erosion	Depressed lesion resulting from loss of epidermis without involvement of dermis
Ulcer	Depressed lesion resulting from loss of epidermis and portion of dermis
Scar	A hard, sclerotic atea of skin after from damage to dermis and subsequent healing
Excoriation	Superficial excavations of skin from scratching
Fissure	Linear cracks in the skin; may be painful
Telangiectasia	Dilated, small blood vessels (capillaries, venules, or arterioles)

Secondary Changes

Erythema	Redness of skin often accompanied by increased temperature, pain, and swelling of skin
Hyperpigmentation	Increase in skin pigment, resulting in darker area of skin
Hypopigmentation	Decrease in skin pigment, resulting in lighter area of skin
Hyperkeratosis	Thickening of stratum corneum
Atrophy	Loss of dermis and/or subcutaneous fat
Exudate	Skin fluid in areas of inflammation, lesions, surgical sites; may be clear, cloudy, or purulent
Crust	Accumulation of dried exudate
Scale	Shedding of outer layer of epidermis (stratum corneum)
Lichenification	Thickened plaques from repeated rubbing or scratching of skin
Purpura	Ecchymotic (dark purple), nonblanching skin lesions from vascular injury and hemorrhage

(Continued)

■ TABLE 1-1 (Continued)	
Distribution	
Localized	Face, neck, chest, abdomen, arm, leg, back, groin
Extensive	Covering several areas of the body
Limited	On only one side of body (e.g., in hair-bearing areas)
Configuration	
Annular	Circular
Annular/central clearing	Circular but clear in center
Linear	In a line
Serpentinus	Snakelike, wavy
Targetoid	Bulls-eye shaped with concentric rings
Grouped	Clustered
Dermatomal	Following a dermatome

■ BOX 1-1 Gram Stain

Smear thin layer of specimen onto glass slide.
Air dry slide; heat fix by running slide above flame (couple of seconds).
Flood slide with crystal violet (10 seconds).
Rinse with water.
Flood with Gram's iodine (10 seconds).
Rinse with water.
Decolorize with acetone (a few seconds).
Rinse with water.
Flood with safarin counterstain (10 seconds).
Rinse with water and air dry.
Note color of bacteria: purple (gram positive) or red (gram negative).
Note arrangement of bacteria: whether found singly, in clusters, in pairs, or in chains.
Note shape of bacteria: round (cocci) or brick-shaped (rods).
Note whether bacteria are located free in the specimen (extracellular) or within cells (intracellular).

---

lesion is dry, use a swab moistened with sterile saline to take the sample. For a fungal culture, put the skin scrapings into a sterile test tube or on Sabouraud's agar for transport to the laboratory. If deep infection is suspected, biopsy is helpful. The sample is bisected vertically: half is sent to the microbiology laboratory for culture, and the other half is sent to pathology for histologic examination.

Biopsies are performed when diagnosis of a skin problem is uncertain. The type and probable depth of a lesion suggests whether shave biopsy, punch biopsy, or incisional or excisional biopsy should be performed (Box 1-2). For each type of biopsy, inform the patient of the procedural risks, give him or her an opportunity to ask questions, and ask the patient to sign a consent form.

■ BOX 1-2 Biopsy

Prepare area for biopsy with alcohol, chlorhexidine (Hibiclens), or 10% providone-iodine (Betadine). Inject the area for biopsy with 1% or 2% xylocaine with or without epinephrine.

Use xylocaine *without* epinephrine for biopsies of fingers, toes, or penis.

For shave biopsy use a No. 15 blade or sterile half of a double-edged razor blade. The nature of the lesion will determine how deep to go to obtain an adequate specimen, but most shave biopsies are superficial into the dermis.

Punch biopsy goes deeper, usually into subcutaneous fat, and is closed with sutures that are removed 1 week later if the biopsy is performed on the face, or 2 weeks later if performed elsewhere. Punches come in a variety of sizes; 4 mm is a common size for most biopsies. Punch biopsies 2 mm or less in size normally do not require suturing. A 4-0 suture is used for closing biopsies on the trunk or extremities; 5-0 or 6-0 suture is used for the face and neck.

Apply antibiotic ointment and bandage.

Instruct patient in wound care: keep wound dry overnight, apply ointment twice a day for a couple of weeks. Instruct patient not to put stress (by exercise, stretching, lifting) on any sutures so that skin will heal more effectively.

Important: **Biopsies should not be performed unless an attending physician is present.**

Examination of skin with a Wood's lamp (long-wave ultraviolet light) is helpful in diagnosing certain conditions. Areas of vitiligo appear bright white under Woods lamp illumination. Areas of hypopigmentation, such as those caused by pityriasis versicolor, appear light, but less bright than vitiligo.

Dermal pigmentation appears similar in intensity to that observed by natural light. Epidermal pigmentation increases to different degrees from that observed in natural light. Microsporum fungal infections within the hair shaft fluoresce green. Erythrasma, skin infection caused by *Corynebacterium minutissimum*, fluoresces coral pink under the Woods lamp. Urine that fluoresces pink under the Woods lamp gives a presumptive diagnosis of porphyria.

Developing a Diagnosis and Treatment Plan

Narrow the diagnosis based on the results of the examination, other clues from the patient, and results of any additional tests performed. Establish a diagnosis and develop a treatment plan. Discuss the diagnosis and plan with the patient, give him or her an educational brochure about the problem if available, and answer any questions. Plan a return visit for the patient as necessary for follow-up. Schedule a full skin examination of the patient at least once a year. Discuss routine skin care, sun protection, and changes to watch for in moles.

The Structure and Function of Normal Skin

Skin is the largest organ of the body. It protects the body and transmits information from the environment to the nervous system. Nerves in skin sense heat, cold, pressure, and pain, and the body reacts. Skin plays an important immune function. Immune cells in skin alert the body to antigens attempting to invade through the skin.

Skin is composed of the *epidermis*, the *basement membrane*, the *dermis*, and *subcutaneous fat*.

Epidermis

The uppermost level of skin is the epidermis. In normal conditions, the epidermis replaces itself about every 4 weeks. The predominant cells of the epidermis are keratinocytes. Within the epidermis are several layers of cells: the basal layer (innermost), spinous layer, granular layer, and the cornified envelope (Box 2-1 and Figure 2-1).

The *basal layer* is the innermost layer of epidermis. New cells (keratinocytes) are born in this layer and travel upward to the skin surface. As new keratinocytes arise from the basal layer, their predecessors are displaced upward toward the skin surface, differentiating along the way. Formation of keratins, proteins important in structural integrity of the cells, begins in the basal layer.

The *spinous layer* is above the basal layer. There spinelike projections, called desmosomes, attach one cell to another. The desmosomes detach and reattach as cells move upward. Gap junctions

---

■ BOX 2-1 The Layers of Skin

1. Epidermis
   Cornified envelope (outermost layer)
   Granular layer
   Spinous layer
   Basal layer (innermost layer)
2. Basement membrane
3. Dermis
   Papillary dermis (outermost layer)
   Reticular dermis (innermost layer)
4. Subcutaneous fat

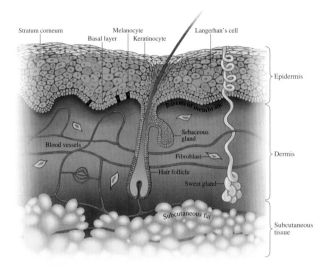

Figure 2-1 • Layers of the skin.

in cell walls allow communication via substances that move in and out of cells. These substances control growth and migration and alert cells to the need for skin repair.

The *granular layer* is above the spinous layer. Here cells develop keratohyalin granules and lamellar bodies in preparation for joining the next layer, the cornified envelope.

The *cornified envelope* is the outermost layer of skin. This layer holds moisture within skin and protects it from the outside environment. A keratinocyte entering the cornified envelope becomes a flattened *corneocyte*, which migrates upward as part of the cornified envelope for approximately 14 days until it is shed.

In addition to keratinocytes, other cells in the epidermis include melanocytes (pigment-producing cells); Langerhan's cells (immune cells); and Merkel's cells (sensory cells).

Melanocytes are responsible for pigmentation of skin and hair. These cells proliferate in response to stimulation by ultraviolet light or inflammatory processes and produce melanin in packets called melanosomes. These melanosomes are transferred to keratinocytes in the lower layers of the epidermis.

In the production of melanin, tyrosine is converted to dopa via tyrosinase. In melanosomes, dopa is transformed into melanin. Differences in distribution of melanosomes within keratinocytes, in size of melanosomes, and in amount and type of melanin produced account for differences in skin color.

Darker skin has larger melanosomes than lighter skin, and melanosomes are dispersed individually throughout the cytoplasm of keratinocytes. In light skin the melanosomes are less dispersed; they are gathered together in membrane-bound groups of melanosomes.

Langerhan's cells are dendritic cells in the epidermis that play an important immune function in skin by detecting antigen, processing the antigen, presenting it to the T cells, and activating the T cells.

Merkel's cells are slow-adapting touch receptors in the epidermis to which unmyelinated, free nerve endings associate. These cells are found in the basal layer of the epidermis and associate with sensory (touch) nerves around hair follicles.

Basement Membrane

The *basement membrane* underlies the basal cell layer and separates the epidermis from the dermis. The basement membrane contains an "anchoring complex" (Figure 2-2) of structures that attach the epidermal cells to the dermis. The anchoring complex extends from hemidesmosomes of basal cells via anchoring filaments through the lamina densa of basement membrane to anchoring fibrils, which encircle collagens in the dermis to form a secure anchor of epidermis, basement membrane, and dermis.

Laminin 5 is a major component of the anchoring filaments. Defects in laminin 5 can result in cicatricial pemphigoid (blistering disorder), in which lack of strong anchoring filaments permits easy separation of epidermis from dermis. Type IV collagen, a major component of the basement membrane of skin as well as the basement membrane of blood vessels and nerves, provides structure and strength to the basement membrane. Anchoring fibrils are

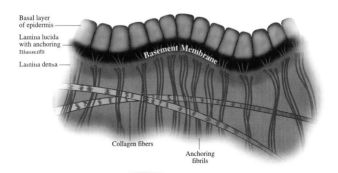

Basal layer of epidermis

Lamina lucida with anchoring filaments

Lamina densa

Basement Membrane

Collagen fibers

Anchoring fibrils

Figure 2-2 • Anchoring complex. Layers of the skin.

composed of type VII collagen. Defects in type VII collagen can result in epidermolysis bullosa (blistering disorder) in which lack of strong anchoring fibrils permits easy separation of epidermis from dermis.

Dermis

The dermis lies below the basement membrane, and can be separated into the upper (papillary) dermis and the lower (reticular) dermis. The dermis consists of connective tissue, cells, and "ground substance" that fill spaces between the connective tissue and cells (Tables 2-1 and 2-2 and Box 2-2). The predominant cells of the dermis are fibroblasts. Fibroblasts circulate through the dermis, producing and degrading connective tissue proteins as necessary.

Connective tissue in the dermis includes collagen and elastic fibers. Collagen is the main structural component of the dermis. Elastic fibers provide skin elasticity. More than 20 collagen types

■ TABLE 2-1 Predominant Collagens in the Dermis

Collagen Type	Location
I	Throughout dermis (80% of collagen in dermis)
III	Throughout dermis (15% of collagen in dermis)
IV	Important component of basement membrane
VI	Found around nerves, blood vessels, and fat cells in dermis
VII	Major component of anchoring fibrils

■ TABLE 2-2 Elastic Fibers in the Dermis

Elaunin fibers	Found in plexus in papillary dermis
Oxytalan fibers	Connect plexus to basement membrane zone
Thick elastic fibers	Found in the deep dermis

■ BOX 2-2 "Ground Substance" in the Dermis

Mucopolysaccharides*
Plasma proteins
Water
Electrolytes

*Mucopolysaccharides are chains of sugar and uronic acid (glycosaminoglycans). These chains link to polypeptides to form proteoglycans. Hyaluronic acid and dermatan sulfate are important glycosaminoglycans in the dermis.

have been discovered in the dermis, with collagens types I and III the predominant types.

Mast cells and small numbers of lymphocytes are also found in the dermis in normal conditions

Mast cells are secretory cells that arise in bone marrow. They synthesize and store mediators such as histamine, heparin, neutrophil chemotactic factor, and eosinophilic chemotactic factor as well as growth factors, cytokines, and platelet-activating factors. Mast cells are responsible for immediate-type hypersensitivity reactions in skin and are involved in chronic inflammatory diseases of the skin. Activated mast cells are important in the skin defense system against parasites and in tumor surveillance.

Lymphocytes are normally found in small numbers in the dermis around blood vessels. In many pathologic conditions, migration of lymphocytes occurs from the blood vessels to dermis, expanding their numbers in the dermis. *T-lymphocytes* defend against intracellular pathogens such as viruses (cellular immunity). *B-lymphocytes* stimulate antibody formation to fight extracellular bacterial, viral, and parasitic infections (humoral immunity) and also play a role in allergic responses. *Natural killer lymphocytes* play a role in nonspecific immune responses to bacteria and viruses. At sites of inflammation they may be joined by leukocytes from the blood.

Other cells found in the dermis include *endothelial cells* (components of blood vessels), *veil cells* and *pericytes* (emcompass blood vessels), and *Schwann's cells* (surround nerve cells). *Monocytes, macrophages*, and *dermal dendritic cells* comprise the phagocytic system of the dermis. Dermal dendritic cells may have an antigen-presenting function in the dermis similar to Langerhan's cells in the epidermis.

The dermis also contains blood vessels, nerves, and specialized structures such as hair follicles, sebaceous glands, and sweat glands.

■ Blood Vessels

Arterioles, venules, and arterial and venous capillaries provide nutrients for the dermis and epidermis and are important in the regulation of temperature control and heat loss. Arterioles and venules form two plexuses in the dermis: the upper plexus (papillary dermis) and the lower plexus (interface of dermis and subcutaneous fat). From the upper plexus, capillary loops rise into the papillary dermis. Arterioles and venules connect the upper and lower plexus and supply sweat glands and hair bulbs.

The majority of vessels in the papillary dermis are postcapillary venules, where inflammatory cells from the blood migrate between the endothelial cells and into the tissues during inflammatory processes. As vessels pass from the deep dermis into the superficial fat, valves are present in the vessels to enhance circulation of blood. Smooth muscle cells and pericytes comprise the contractile elements in the microvasculature.

■ Nerves

Sensations of temperature, pressure, pain, and touch are detected by sensory nerves in skin and transmitted to the central nervous system. Motor (effector) nerves in skin innervate blood vessels (to effect vasoconstriction), sweat glands (to effect sweating), and the arrector pili muscle that attaches to hair follicles (to cause "goose bumps"). Neuropeptides allow communication between nerves and skin cells (including immune cells). Sensory nerves in the dermis include *Pacinian corpuscles* (vibration), *Meissner's corpuscles* (touch), *Ruffini's corpuscles* (pressure), and *Krause's endbulbs* (sensory in mucous membranes).

■ Specialized Structures

Specialized structures in the dermis include hair follicles, sebaceous glands, eccrine (sweat) glands, and apocrine (sweat) glands.

A *hair follicle* is depicted in Figure 2-3. Signals between epidermis and dermis are important in the continuous hair cycle of growth and rest. The dermal papilla at the base of the hair follicle plays an important role in stimulating anagen, or the growth phase of the hair cycle. The dermal papilla contains blood vessels, dermal papilla cells, and extracellular matrix. Above the dermal papilla at the base of the hair follicle is the hair matrix, which gives rise to a hair from rapidly dividing cells in the matrix. The hair follicle encloses the hair, as it grows, with both an outer root sheath and an inner root sheath. The inner root sheath molds the shape of the hair and has three layers from innermost outward: the *cuticle, Huxley's layer*, and *Henle's layer*. The cuticle surrounds the hair, its cells overlapping like roof tiles. The cortex of the hair is composed of long, narrow, closely packed cortical cells containing keratin filaments. Inside the cortex is the medulla, the inner core of hair. The medulla consists of spongelike keratin and amorphous material. Hair follicles originate and cycle through anagen (growth), catagen (regression), and telogen (resting) phases of the hair cycle. Hormones, enzymes, androgens, and other factors affect hair growth. Scientists continue to work to understand the elusive mechanisms of hair growth.

Sebaceous glands are found primarily on the face and secrete lipids that provide lubrication for facial skin. These glands are located in the dermis, with ducts leading to the surface that are also shared by hair follicles. Sebum from sebaceous glands travels upward through the sebaceous duct, lined by squamous cells, and through the follicular infundibulum (extends from the opening of the sebaceous duct into the hair follicle canal [pilar canal] to

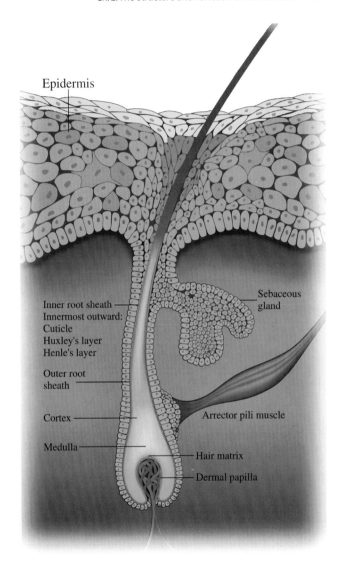

Figure 2-3 · Hair follicle.

the skin surface). Overactivity of sebaceous glands, stimulated by hormones during puberty, can precipitate acne.

Eccrine glands are sweat glands found on all parts of the body. They are important in regulating body temperature. These glands are stimulated by temperature and emotion.

Sweat is formed by secretion of a plasmalike fluid containing sodium chloride (NaCl). NaCl is then reabsorbed from the fluid in the sweat duct. Sweat flows from the secretory gland through a coiled duct and then into a straight intradermal duct that connects to a spiraled intraepidermal duct leading to the skin surface.

Apocrine glands differ in function and composition from eccrine glands. Commonly found in axilla, buttocks, groin, and scalp, their primary function appears to be production of scent. Scent production is achieved through apocrine secretion (pinching off apical portions of apocrine cells containing secretory granules). A milky substance is produced and stored to be released intermittently through apocrine ducts that open into the follicular infundibula or directly onto the skin surface.

Subcutaneous Fat

The *subcutaneous fat* lies between the dermis above and fascia below. It serves as a thermal and mechanical buffer zone for the internal organs. Between fat lobules are fibrous septa that contain blood vessels, nerves, and lymphatics. Blood vessels send out small branches to form capillaries that surround each fat cell, and they also send larger branches up into the deep vascular plexus of the dermis.

3 Disorders of Structure and Function

DISORDERS OF THE STRATUM CORNEUM AND UPPER LAYERS OF THE EPIDERMIS

Damage to the cornified envelope can occur from the external environment, resulting in disruption of the barrier function of skin and stimulation of cytokine production.

- Results in skin dryness (xerosis) and cracking (fissuring), itching (pruritus), redness (erythema), and scaling.
- Barrier disruption can also occur from intrinsic defects such as essential fatty acid deficiency, which leads to insufficient lipid deposition in the stratum corneum.
- Treatment includes protection against water loss from skin by use of moisturizers (unscented) applied immediately after bathing (pat dry the skin and then immediately apply). Mild, unscented soap should be used for bathing.
- Barrier disruption can also occur from other scaling disorders such as pityriasis rosea and psoriasis.

SCALING ERUPTIONS

Pityriasis Rosea (Figure 3-1)

■ **Definition**
- Papulosquamous eruption

■ **Etiology**
- Cause unknown

■ **Appearance**
- Widespread, usually involving trunk and extremities
- Disease self-limited
- Usually starts with an erythematous, annular, scaling plaque, called a "herald patch" (see Figure 3-1) that is followed a couple of weeks later by a generalized papulosquamous eruption (slightly raised papules or plaques) on the trunk and proximal extremities.

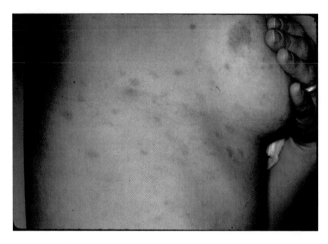

Figure 3-1 • Pityriasis rosea. *(Image courtesy of Dr. Howard Baden, Massachusetts General Hospital/Harvard Medical School, Boston, MA.)*

■ Diagnosis

• Because secondary syphilis can be confused with pityriasis rosea, obtain serology to rule out syphilis.

■ Treatment

• Treatment normally not indicated. If itching is present, oral antihistamine can be helpful.

Psoriasis (Figure 3-2)

■ Definition

• Chronic disorder characterized by plaques with erythema and scale.

■ Etiology

• Etiology unknown.
• Occurs equally in males and females.
• Guttate psoriasis sometimes develops following throat infection with streptococcus; superantigens may therefore be involved.
• Genetic predisposition appears to exist.
• Environmental factors appear to play a precipitating role.
• Patients often feel that stress exacerbates their condition.

■ Appearance

• Plaques often found on the elbows, knees, lower back, and scalp, but can involve all parts of the body.

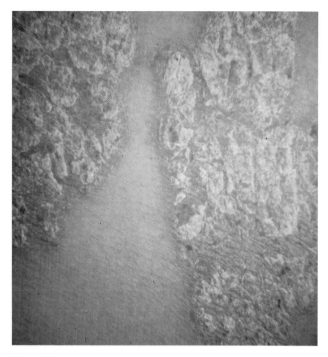

Figure 3-2 • Psoriasis. *(Image courtesy of Dr. Howard Baden, Massachusetts General Hospital/Harvard Medical School, Boston, MA.)*

- Can also present as a generalized erythroderma (redness of skin all over), a pustular eruption (von Zumbusch's pustular psoriasis), and a guttate eruption (small plaques over trunk and proximal extremities).
- The Koebner's phenomenon (new psoriatic lesions arise at the site of trauma) characteristic.
- Inverse psoriasis involves plaques in the groin, axilla, submammary areas, navel, and intergluteal fold.
- Psoriasis can also affect nails and joints (psoriatic arthritis).
- Nail changes may include yellow-brown discoloration, pitting, misshapen nails (onychodystrophy), and separation of the nail from the nail bed (onycholysis).

■ **Diagnosis**
- Biopsy and clinical appearance can confirm diagnosis.

■ **Treatment**
- Sunshine and ocean bathing still valid treatments.
- Topical tar preparations or topical tar plus ultraviolet B.

- Topical corticosteroids (bid medium strength), topical tazarotene (retinoid), coal tar, anthralin, or oral or topical vitamin D analogues such as calcitriol and calcipotriol.
- Daily use of unscented moisturizers important.
- Avoidance of perfumed soaps and perfumed lotions.
- Methotrexate, PUVA (psoralens, which are orally administered photosensitizing substances, plus ultraviolet A irradiation), or oral retinoids such as acitretin can be helpful for more severe cases with widespread lesions.
- Narrow-band ultraviolet B irradiation can be very helpful, as can combinations of retinoids plus PUVA, or retinoids and ultraviolet B irradiation.
- Topical or oral cyclosporine has also been used to treat psoriasis.

ECZEMATOUS ERUPTIONS

Eczema (Figure 3-3)

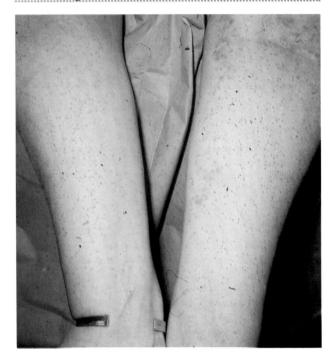

Figure 3-3 • Eczema. *(Image courtesy of Dr. Howard Baden, Massachusetts General Hospital/Harvard Medical School, Boston, MA.)*

See also the section on Atopic Dermatitis in Chapter 6.

■ **Definition**
- Chronic disorder characterized by erythema, scale, and sometimes crusting and oozing.
- Conditions that resemble eczema are characterized as eczematous eruptions and include seborrheic dermatitis, lichen simplex chronicus, and contact dermatitis.

■ **Etiology**
- *Eczema* is a general term sometimes used to refer to atopic dermatitis, but also to other conditions caused by irritation of skin by scratching or by a variety of substances, such as perfumed lotions or soaps, dish detergent, or exposure to other irritants or allergans.
- Colonization of chronic eczema with bacteria sometimes occurs, and lichenification (thickening) of skin can occur with scratching.

■ **Appearance**
- Plaques and patches with erythema, scale, crusting, oozing

■ **Diagnosis**
- Biopsy if diagnosis is unclear
- Culture of specific, persistent lesions

■ **Treatment**
- Topical corticosteroids or topical tacrolimus.
- Important to emphasize importance of mild, unscented soaps and unscented moisturizers; avoidance of irritating substances in daily skin care.
- Antibiotics sometimes necessary to treat flares.

Seborrheic Dermatitis (Figure 3-4)

■ **Definition**
- Common disorder characterized by plaques and patches with erythema and scale.

■ **Etiology**
- The cause of seborrheic dermatitis is unknown, although the lipophilic yeast *Pityrosporum ovale* may play a role.
- Babies as well as adults are affected.
- Occurs in areas that correspond to general locations of sebaceous glands; however, seborrheic dermatitis is not thought to be due to dysfunction of the sebaceous glands.

■ **Appearance**
- "Cradle cap" (Figure 3-5), characterized by plaques and scale on the scalp of babies, is a form of seborrheic dermatitis.

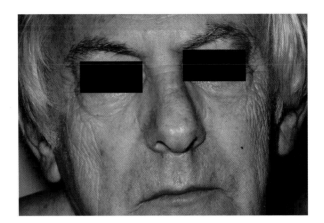

Figure 3-4 • Seborrheic dermatitis. *(Image courtesy of Dr. Howard Baden, Massachusetts General Hospital/Harvard Medical School, Boston, MA.)*

- In adults, seborrheic dermatitis is usually found as scale and erythema in the nasolabial folds, postauricular area, malar area (across cheeks and bridge of nose), anterior chest, middle back, and scalp, as well as flaking in the eyebrows.

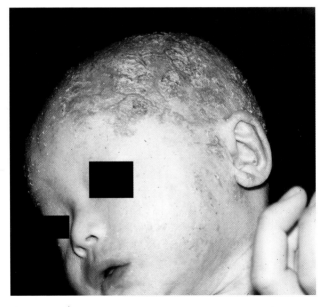

Figure 3-5 • Cradle cap. *(Image courtesy of Dr. Howard Baden, Massachusetts General Hospital/Harvard Medical School, Boston, MA.)*

- Histopathology: spongiosis (collection of fluid between individual keratinocytes) and infiltration of lymphocytes around vessels of the superficial plexus.

■ **Diagnosis**
- Diagnosis can usually be made by clinical appearance and areas of involvement.
- Although seborrheic dermatitis is a common condition, sudden onset of seborrheic dermatitis or psoriasis should prompt investigation of underlying HIV infection.

■ **Treatment**
- Seborrheic dermatitis responds to medications that inhibit growth of yeast, including topical ketoconazole and selenium sulfide.
- Treatment of seborrheic dermatitis of the scalp includes medicated shampoo (containing ingredients such as zinc pyrithione, selenium sulfide, ketoconazole, glycolic acid, salicylic acid, or tar).
- Topical steroid solutions can be used twice a day on the scalp for resistant areas.
- Topical mild corticosteroids may be used on the face for a few days if inflammation is significant, but anti-yeast medication should be first-line treatment.

Lichen Simplex Chronicus (Figure 3-6)

■ **Definition**
- Common disorder characterized by plaques with erythema, skin lichenification (thickening), and scale

■ **Etiology**
- Cause: chronic scratching of skin.
- Lesions are extremely pruritic (itchy), and patients scratch vigorously, causing increase in itching and skin damage and continuation of the itch/scratch cycle.

■ **Appearance**
- Lesions are usually localized in places easy to scratch, such as lower legs or upper arms. Secondary infection often occurs.
- Histopathology: epidermal hyperplasia (thickened epidermis) and thickened bundles of collagen in the upper dermis.

■ **Diagnosis**
- Diagnosis is usually made by clinical appearance.
- Biopsy if diagnosis uncertain.

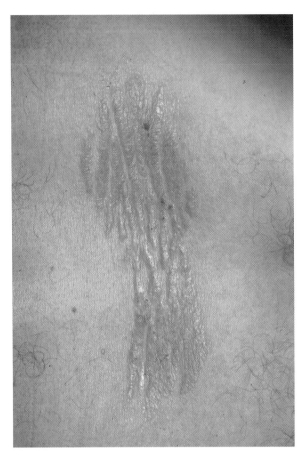

Figure 3-6 • Lichen simplex chronicus. *(Image courtesy of Dr. Howard Baden, Massachusetts General Hospital/Harvard Medical School, Boston, MA.)*

■ Treatment
• Treatment is topical steroids, cessation of scratching, antihistamines if necessary to reduce itching, and antibiotics if superimposed infection is suspected.

PUSTULAR DISORDERS

Candida albicans Infection (Figure 3-7)

■ Definition
• Pustular eruption caused by the yeast *Candida albicans*

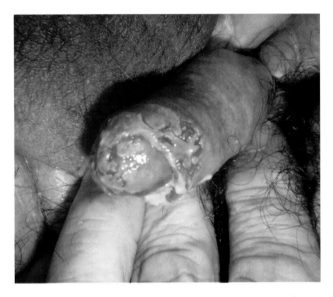

Figure 3-7 • *Candida albicans. (Image courtesy of Dr. Howard Baden, Massachusetts General Hospital/Harvard Medical School, Boston, MA.)*

■ Etiology

- Infection with the yeast *Candida albicans*
- Yeast organisms found normally in the mouth, gastrointestinal tract, and vaginal mucosa cause disease when they proliferate and invade the skin or mucous membranes (especially in the setting of immunosuppression, pregnancy, diabetes, or antibiotic therapy).
- Can also occur as diaper dermatitis.
- Can be cause of nail disease with distal onycholysis (separation of the nail) and white discoloration.

■ Appearance

- Bright pink erythema with pustules and scale, often under the breasts or in the groin.
- Lesions usually well demarcated, but satellite lesions of pustules and erythema with less well-defined borders often occur.
- Mucocutaneous disease (vaginitis, balantis, oral candidiasis [thrush]): yellow-white plaques or white, cheesy deposits.
- Histopathology: spongiform pustular dermatitis, mycelia, and yeast in stratum corneum; neutrophils in upper spinous and granular layers.

■ **Diagnosis**

• Diagnosis often based on clinical appearance; can be confirmed by skin scrapings and culture that show yeast forms producing germ tubes.

• In systemic candidiasis, mycelia and yeast are present in the dermis and walls of blood vessels.

■ **Treatment**

• Clotrimazole (topical, oral, or vaginal; e.g., Lotrimin), itraconazole (oral; e.g., Sporonox), ketoconazole (topical or oral; e.g., Nizoral), nystatin (oral/topical/vaginal; e.g., Mycostatin), fluconazole (oral; e.g., Diflucan), and miconazole (vaginal; e.g., Monistat)

• Oral candidiasis: mycelex troches or nystatin swish and spit preparations

• Intertriginous candidiasis: topical ketoconazole

• Vaginal candidiasis: oral diflucan

CYSTIC DISORDERS

Epidermal Cyst (Figure 3-8)

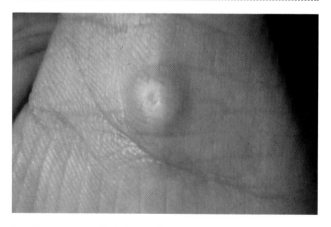

Figure 3-8 • Epidermal inclusion cyst. *(Image courtesy of Dr. Howard Baden, Massachusetts General Hospital/Harvard Medical School, Boston, MA.)*

■ **Definition**

• Keratin-containing cyst lined by stratified squamous cells

■ **Etiology**

• Proliferation of surface epithelial cells within dermis

■ **Appearance**
- Dome-shaped, mobile protuberance of skin
- Sometimes with central punctum
- Contains cheesy, keratinaceous material within cyst wall of stratified squamous cells with granular cell layer

■ **Diagnosis**
- Clinical appearance

■ **Treatment**
- No treatment necessary unless inflamed or otherwise troublesome
- If inflamed: incision, drainage, antibiotics
- After inflammation subsides, excision to remove remaining cyst and epidermal lining

Milia

■ **Definition**
- Tiny keratin-filled cysts that occur singly or in multiples on the face

■ **Etiology**
- Arise *de novo* or as a result of trauma
- Commonly occur in the epidermis
- Hereditary component in some cases of multiple milia

■ **Appearance**
- Whitish papules on face

■ **Diagnosis**
- None usually necessary

■ **Treatment**
- If troublesome to the patient, can be removed by incision and removal of the contents.

DISORDERS OF SKIN APPENDAGES

- Include sebaceous glands, eccrine glands, apocrine glands, and hair.
- Disorders can result from hyperactivity, hypoactivity, or occlusion or malfunction of normal skin appendages or from abnormal skin appendages.

Acne (Figure 3-9)

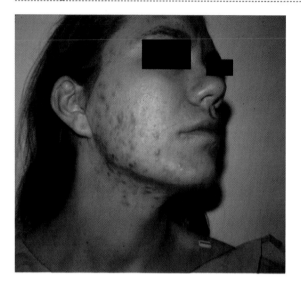

Figure 3-9 • Acne. *(Image courtesy of Dr. Howard Baden, Massachusetts General Hospital/Harvard Medical School, Boston, MA.)*

■ **Definition**

• Acne: skin condition characterized by pustules, erythematous papules, sebaceous cysts, comedones, and inflammation.

■ **Etiology**

• Precipitated by several factors affecting the pilosebaceous unit.
• The pilosebaceous unit consists of sebaceous glands surrounding hair follicles on the face, back, upper arms, and chest.
• Most common during teen years, but also can occur in adulthood.
• Pathophysiology: (1) sebaceous glands stimulated by circulating androgens to produce excessive sebum (triglycerides, wax esters, squalene, cholesterol, and cholesterol esters); (2) hypercornification (thickening of wall) of the pilosebaceous duct (pilar canal), blocking effective secretion of sebum; (3) increased colonization of the pilosebaceous duct (passageway for sebum to skin surface) with bacteria, commonly *Propionibacterium acnes*, which break down free fatty acids in sebum into inflammatory substances.
• Risk factors for acne: hereditary, certain medications, such as lithium steroids.
• In females often worse around time of menstrual period.

- Neonatal acne (Figure 3-10) occasionally seen in newborns for first 2 to 3 weeks after birth, caused by passage of maternal hormones through the placenta.

■ **Appearance**

- Eruption of inflammatory papules, pustules on face, may be on upper arms, chest, and back.
- Common lesions include papules, pustules, comedones, scarring, cysts, and erythema.
- In adult acne, cysts tend to occur on the lower jaw, chin, and neck and in females often correlate in occurrence with the menstrual period.
- Acne cysts may result in scarring.

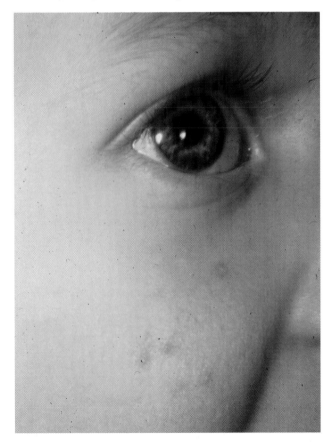

Figure 3-10 • Acne neonatorum. *(Image courtesy of Dr. Howard Baden, Massachusetts General Hospital/Harvard Medical School, Boston, MA.)*

■ **Diagnosis**
- Check DHEAS, free testosterone in severe cases of female acne

■ **Treatment**
- Topical: for predominant lesions of inflammatory papules, pustules, and comedones
  - Erythromycin or clindamycin qam.
  - Tretinoin (Retin A), adapalene (Differin), azelaic acid (Azelex), or benzoyl peroxide cream or gel qpm.
  - Benzoyl peroxide or salicylic acid wash can be useful if facial skin is oily, also useful in treating acne on back, upper arms, and chest. Apply in shower and rinse well. *Caution:* **Can bleach clothes if not rinsed well from skin.**
- Oral: Acne with inflammatory cysts may require one of the following oral medications:
  - Tetracycline 500 mg bid
  - Minocycline 100 mg bid
  - Doxycycline 100 mg qd or bid
  - Erythromycin 500 mg bid
- *Caution:* **Tetracycline or its analogues (minocycline, doxycycline) should not be used in patients under 11 years of age or in pregnant women since it can cause yellowing of the developing teeth of children and fetuses.**
- Severe cases with scarring and cysts may require consideration of isotretinoin (Accutane). *Caution:* **Isotretinoin can cause severe birth defects and other serious side effects. Strict protocols, including two forms of birth control in females of child-bearing age, must be followed.**

Pilar (trichilemmal) Cyst (Figure 3-11)

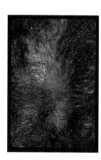

Figure 3-11 • Pilar cyst. *(Image courtesy of Dr. Howard Baden, Massachusetts General Hospital/Harvard Medical School, Boston, MA.)*

■ **Definition**
- Keratin-containing cyst lined by epithelium resembling outer root sheath of hair

■ Etiology
• Often autosomal-dominant inheritance

■ Appearance
• Dome-shaped, mobile protuberance, usually on scalp
• Contains keratinaceous material; no granular cell layer present in cyst wall

■ Diagnosis
• Clinical appearance

■ Treatment
• No treatment necessary unless inflamed or otherwise troublesome
• Excision if troublesome

Sebaceous Hyperplasia (Figure 3-12)

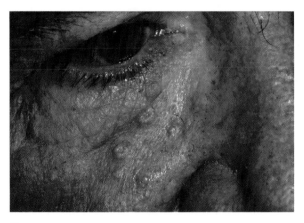

Figure 3-12 • Sebaceous hyperplasia. *(Image courtesy of Dr. Howard Baden, Massachusetts General Hospital/Harvard Medical School, Boston, MA.)*

■ Definition
• Common condition in adults characterized by enlargement of sebaceous glands on forehead and cheeks of middle-aged or older individuals.

■ Etiology
• Unknown, possible genetic influence

■ Appearance
• Yellowish or flesh-colored papules with central umbilication

■ **Diagnosis**
• Biopsy if it cannot be distinguished clinically from skin carcinoma

■ **Treatment**
• Of no consequence except for cosmetic concerns
• Can be removed by light electrodessication

Rhinophyma (Figure 3-13)

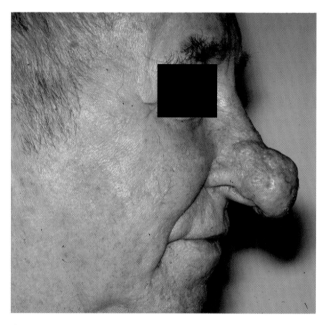

Figure 3-13 • Rhinophyma. *(Image courtesy of Dr. Howard Baden, Massachusetts General Hospital/Harvard Medical School, Boston, MA.)*

■ **Definition**
• Enlargement of the sebaceous glands resulting in bulbous nose

■ **Etiology**
• Sometimes seen in men over 40 with rosacea
• Cause unknown

■ **Appearance**
• Nose: hypertrophy of soft tissues of the nose with inflammatory nodules, dilated pores with large plugs of sebum and

keratin; often distortion of the nose by lobular masses of sebaceous tissue

- Histologically: hypertrophy of sebaceous glands and fibrosis of dermis

■ **Treatment**

- Surgical shaving of the nose.
- Tetracycline 500 mg po bid may be helpful in preventing further hypertrophy.

DISORDERS OF ECCRINE SWEAT GLANDS

Hyperhidrosis

■ **Definition**

- Excessive sweat production by eccrine glands, often involving palms, soles, and axillae.

■ **Etiology**

- Genetic tendency likely in many cases.
- Heat or emotional stimuli can stimulate excessive sweating.
- Neurologic, vascular, metabolic, or infectious disorders stimulate excessive sweating.

■ **Appearance**

- Excess sweat production involves palms, soles, and axillae.
- Sweaty handshakes and drenching of clothes at business meetings or social functions.

■ **Treatment**

- Topical antiperspirants
- For more severe cases, the following may be tried:
  - Oral anticholinergic medications if problem severe. **Caution: Systemic side effects of anticholinergic medications include loss of urinary bladder spincter control, dry mouth, dry eyes, and decreased gastric peristalsis.**
  - Surgical excision of axillae vault. **Caution: Significant scarring can result.**
  - Liposuction of sweat glands.
  - Water iontophoresis-induced inhibition of sweating of palms and sole. **Note: Requires treatment of each palm or sole for approximately half an hour each day with an iontophoresis unit.**
  - Injection of botulinum toxin into palms or soles. **Important: Must be performed by a physician experienced in this technique.**

- *Note:* Other disorders of sweat glands include anhidrosis (absence of sweating), and hypohidrosis (decreased sweating).

DISORDERS OF APOCRINE SWEAT GLANDS

Hidradenitis Suppurativa (Figure 3-14)

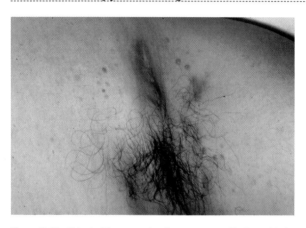

Figure 3-14 • Hidradenitis suppurativa. *(Image courtesy of Dr. Howard Baden, Massachusetts General Hospital/Harvard Medical School, Boston, MA.)*

■ **Definition**
- Chronic, suppurative disease of apocrine sweat gland areas

■ **Etiology**
- Keratinaceous occlusion of apocrine ducts and secondary bacterial infection
- Bacteria breakdown of secretory products into fatty acid molecules, producing characteristic odor

■ **Appearance**
- Inflammatory nodules, cysts with suppuration, and scarring in apocrine gland areas.
- Sinus tract formation and fibrosis common

■ **Diagnosis**
- Diagnosis usually made by location and appearance of lesions.
- Culture may be done if secondary infection suspected.

■ **Treatment**
- Topical and oral antibiotics (erythromycin, tetracycline, minocycline, or cephalosporins).

- Long-term therapy may be necessary.
- Surgical excision of involved areas can be effective in severe cases.
- *Note*: **Other disorders of apocrine sweat glands include hydrocystomas and apocrine carcinomas.**

DISORDERS OF THE HAIR FOLLICLE

Folliculitis (Figure 3-15)

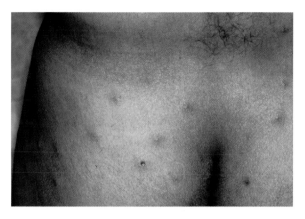

Figure 3-15 • Folliculitis. *(Image courtesy of Dr. Howard Baden, Massachusetts General Hospital/Harvard Medical School, Boston, MA.)*

■ **Definition**
- Irritation of hair follicles, resulting in perifollicular inflammation and papular or pustular formation on the skin surface

■ **Etiology**
- Trauma to hair follicles from clothes rubbing against skin or from sweating while exercising
- Steroids
- Antineoplastic agents (actinomycin D, methotrexate)
- Yeast infections (e.g., *Pityrosporum* folliculitis caused by the yeast *Malassezia furfur*)
- Bacterial infections (e.g., *Pseudomonas* folliculitis often occurs after bathing in hot tubs)
- Other infections

■ **Appearance**
- Perifollicular papules with erythema.

- *Pityrisporum* folliculitis, caused by the yeast *Malassezia furfur*, usually occurs on the back, chest, and upper extremities and causes inflammatory papules or pustules. *Pityrisporum* folliculitis is usually very pruritic (itchy).
- *Pseudomonas* folliculitis causes erythematous papules, pustules, macules, and vesicles.

■ Diagnosis
- Usually diagnosed by clinical appearance and history
- Skin scraping and Gram stain, culture, or biopsy if in doubt

■ Treatment
- Benzoyl peroxide wash used in the shower to affected areas. *Caution:* **Rinse well, since residual benzoyl peroxide can bleach clothes.**
- Mild keratolytic preparations such as ammonium lactate moisturizer applied to affected areas.
- *Pityrosporum* folliculitis can be treated with topical ketoconazole or topical application of 2.5% selenium sulfide solution.
- "Hot tub folliculitis": Use benzoyl peroxide wash in the shower to the affected areas and then rinse off. For severe, recalcitrant cases with systemic symptoms, ciprofloxacin 500 mg bid can be prescribed.

DISORDERS OF HAIR GROWTH

Hair growth is a cyclic process that involves a growth phase (anagen) that usually lasts several years, a transitional or involutional phase (catagen) that lasts a few days to a few weeks, and a resting phase (telogen) that lasts a few weeks to a few months. Hair is then shed, and the anagen phase resumes with development of a new hair. The hair growth cycle in humans is not synchronized, so that all of the hairs do not go through anagen, catagen, and telogen simultaneously. Thus, we do not usually notice the shedding process other than finding hairs in our hairbrush.

Alopecia

■ Definition
- Loss of hair (too little hair growth or balding)

■ Etiology
- Aging: androgen-dependent conversion of regular scalp hair into vellus, or very fine, light, short hairs.
- Genetic disorders: Hereditary syndromes characterized by alopecia are numerous.

- Immune disregulation
- Hormonal abnormalities: thyroid dysfunction, excessive circulating androgens.
- Medications
- Infections: Syphilis can result in thinning of hair ("moth-eaten alopecia").
- Nutritional deficiencies
- Chemotherapy
- Trauma (pulling hair into pony tails, twirling hair around finger, excessive hair curling)
- Stress
- Certain scalp conditions (e.g., seborrheic dermatitis or psoriasis)
- Many other conditions of uncertain origin.

■ **Appearance**

- Loss of hair
- Alopecia (either scarring or nonscarring). Nonscarring conditions have better chance of improving than scarring conditions.
- Alopecia areata is condition of unknown etiology characterized by well-demarcated patches of alopecia. If entire scalp is involved, it is called alopecia totalis; if generalized body hair is also lost, it is called alopecia universalis.
- Histologically: lymphocytic inflitrate around hair bulbs, suggesting defects in immune regulation leading to autoimmunity

■ **Diagnosis**

- Examine scalp for any abnormalities.
- Perform loose hair pull and examine hairs under a microscope to determine what type of hairs are falling out. Usually telogen hairs (telogen effluvium) will predominate in the hairs that come out easily upon gently pulling scalp hairs. If the loose hairs coming out are in the anagen phase (anagen effluvium), consider one of the medications taken by the patient as the precipitating cause.
- Thyroid function tests
- RPR for syphilis
- DHEAS and free and bound testosterone to detect excessive circulating androgens.
- Punch biopsy of scalp can determine whether scarring is present and whether immune cell infiltration is present. Biopsy also provides information about percentage of anagen, catagen, and telogen hairs in the sample.
- In children, suspect fungal infection as cause of scalp flaking and examine scrapings and hairs under the microscope for fungal hyphae. When in doubt, send fresh specimens to the laboratory for fungal culture.

■ **Treatment**
- Treat underlying cause if cause determined and can be treated.
- The patient with hair loss should be counseled to treat hair gently, and to avoid twisting or pulling hair or combing hair vigorously when wet.
- If fungal infection present, treat with oral antifungal medication. Scalp flaking due to seborrheic dermatitis or psoriasis should be treated with medicated shampoo containing sulfur, zinc, or salicylic acid.

Hypertrichosis

■ **Definition**
- Increase in hair on the body

■ **Etiology**
- May be genetic in origin or acquired.
- May be a result of an underlying disorder, or may be a purely cosmetic concern.
- Excessive hair growth on the midline of the back can sometimes signal congenital nonfusion (dysraphism) of the spine.
- Central nervous system disorders can result in acquired hypertrichosis.
- Can be locally acquired as a result of dermal inflammation from trauma or a variety of skin disorders.
- Can be a side effect of medications.
- Is a feature of many medical syndromes.

■ **Appearance**
- Increased hair on body: may be localized to certain areas of the body or generalized

■ **Diagnosis**
- Acquired hypertrichosis should prompt investigation of underlying medical problems.
- Rapid growth of fine hair all over the body is sometimes associated with carcinoma tumors, lymphomas, and malignancies of the breast, ovary, gallbladder, colon, rectum, uterus, pancreas, and bronchus.

■ **Treatment**
- If treatment of underlying problem is successful, hypertrichosis will often resolve.
- Localized areas of hypertrichosis can be treated with electrolysis, wax epilation, bleaching, shaving, or laser treatment. ***Caution:*** **These methods often cause side effects of skin irritation. Electrolysis and laser hair removal can permanently destroy hair if**

the dermal papilla of the hair follicle is destroyed, but many treatments are usually necessary.

Hirsutism

■ **Definition**
- Androgen-responsive hair growth on females in pattern more typical of that on males.

■ **Etiology**
- Can occur with increased production of androgens, when hormone precursors converted to androgens, when free androgen is elevated because androgen binding proteins are depressed, or when there is increased end-organ sensitivity to androgens. In some hirsute females no underlying endocrinologic disorder is found.
- Can be associated with medications or with ovarian or adrenal disorders that result in hyperprolactinemia and acromegaly. Polycystic ovary syndrome results in anovulation, hyperadrogenism, and hirsutism.

■ **Appearance**
- Hair growth on female in areas such as moustache and beard regions, lower abdomen, chest

■ **Diagnosis**
- Testosterone concentrations in polycystic ovary syndrome patients usually slightly elevated, serum LH levels usually high, FSH concentrations usually low.
- Laboratory tests useful in evaluating hirsutism include serum unbound testosterone, DHEAS, LH/FSH hormone ratio, and prolactin.

■ **Treatment**
- Evaluate for potential underlying problems.
- Same cosmetic procedures described for treatment of hypertrichosis may be useful.
- Medications to block androgen receptors (spironolactone or cyproterone acetate with ethinyl estradiol) helpful in some cases.

DISORDERS OF MELANIN AND MELANOCYTES

- Vitiligo, hypopigmentation, hyperpigmentation
- Melanocytes are cells in the basal layer of skin that produce melanin for protection of skin from ultraviolet radiation.
- Melanocytes make melanin with the help of the enzyme tyrosinase.
- Melanocytes deposit melanin in skin keratinocytes, darkening

the skin to different degrees, depending on the type and amount of pigment produced.

- Many skin disorders are associated with depigmentation or hypopigmentation. Such disorders include lupus erythematosus, cutaneous T-cell lymphoma, scleroderma, and piebaldism (genetic disorder with absence of melanocytes in skin and hair).

Vitiligo (Figure 3-16)

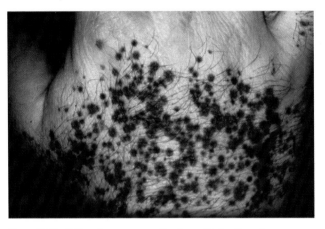

Figure 3-16 • Vitiligo. *(Image courtesy of Dr. Howard Baden, Massachusetts General Hospital/Harvard Medical School, Boston, MA.)*

■ Definition
- Total loss of pigmentation in area(s) of skin
- Melanocytes lost from the epidermis; no melanin produced

■ Etiology
- No established precipitating causes of vitiligo, but there often appears to be a genetic component.
- Destruction of melanocytes, causing white patches of vitiligo, may result from intrinsic dysfunction of melanocytes, chemical toxicity, or autoimmune-mediated destruction.

■ Appearance
- Stark white patches of skin with distinct borders.
- Patches can be localized or extensive.

■ Diagnosis
- Biopsy of a patch of vitiligo shows no melanocytes.

■ Treatment

• Repigmentation requires repopulation with melanocytes. Repopulation of melanocytes can occur by migration of melanocytes from around hair follicles in nearby normal skin.

• Any underlying condition associated with vitiligo must be addressed.

• Patient often concerned primarily for cosmetic reasons.

• Topical steroids can sometimes be helpful for treatment of limited areas of vitiligo.

• Psoralens (given orally or applied topically) and ultraviolet light exposure (PUVA) may be helpful. *Caution:* **The patient undergoing PUVA treatment must avoid sun exposure to skin and eyes, even through a car window, on the day of treatment. Patients should have regular eye examinations. The risk for skin cancers is increased in patients who have had many PUVA treatments.**

• Surgical placement of small minigrafts of normal skin into nonpigmented areas to provide more melanocytes for migration to repigment areas of vitiligo.

Hypomelanosis (Hypopigmentation) and Amelanosis

■ Definition

• Hypomelanosis: decrease in melanin production in skin

• Amelanosis: complete absence of melanin production in skin

■ Etiology

• Hypopigmentation can occur because the number of melanocytes producing melanin decreases or because there is a decrease in the ability of the melanocytes to produce melanin.

• Common causes of hypopigmentation: skin irritation and inflammatory disorders (atopic dermatitis, other skin rashes).

• Either postinflammatory hypopigmentation or hyperpigmentation can occur after inflammatory conditions.

• Common cause of hypopigmentation (and sometimes hyperpigmentation) is pityriasis versicolor, caused by the lipophilic yeast *Malassezia furfur* (*Pityrosporum orbiculare*), which produces azelaic acid, an inhibitor of tyrosinase.

• Many genetic disorders are associated with hypomelanosis or amelanosis:
  - Oculocutaneous albinism: reduced or absent melanin production, resulting in decreased or absent pigmentation of eyes, hair, and skin. There are a variety of clinical manifestations in this condition, resulting from different defects in the tyrosinase gene.

- Hypomelanosis of Ito: multiple streaks of hypopigmentation (reduction in melanin and reduced or normal melanocytes); neurologic, musculoskeletal, and ocular abnormalities.
- Tuberous sclerosis: multiple hypopigmented macules (decrease in pigment, decreased number of melanosomes in melanocytes), multiple facial angiofibromas, multiple ungual fibromas, and cardiac rhabdomyomas
- Waardenburg's syndrome: white forelock and piebaldism (no melanocytes or melanin), dystopia canthorum, broad nasal root, confluent eyebrows, heterochromia irides, and congenital hearing loss.

■ **Appearance**
- Hypopigmentation: less pigmentation than normal for an individual (areas of lighter color than surrounding skin)

■ **Diagnosis**
- If pityriasis versicolor (yeast) is suspected, examine skin scrapings microscopically. Look for yeast forms and short hyphae ("spaghetti and meatballs" appearance).

■ **Treatment**
- Postinflammatory hypopigmentation will usually resolve over time. Avoid skin irritation.
- If hypopigmentation is caused by pityriasis versicolor, treat area with ketoconazole cream applied twice a day or with selenium sulfide lotion (Selsun lotion) 2.5% applied from the neck down, left on overnight, and washed off the following morning. Repeat treatment 1 week later.

Hyperpigmentation

■ **Definition**
- More pigmentation than normal for an individual

■ **Etiology/Pathophysiology**
- Increased melanin distributed in basal layer of epidermis and in macrophages in dermis.
- Results from increased melanin in melanocytes and keratinocytes in basal layer of skin (brown hyperpigmentation) or from macrophages in the dermis that contain melanin (slate gray to blue pigmentation of skin).
- Hyperpigmentation following inflammatory conditions (postinflammatory hyperpigmentation): Inflammatory conditions may decrease melanocyte activity, resulting in skin hypopigmentation, or inflammatory conditions may stimulate melanocytes to increase production of melanin, resulting in skin hyperpigmentation.

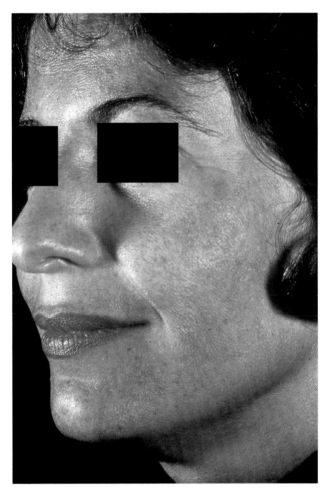

Figure 3-17 • Melasma. *(Image courtesy of Dr. Howard Baden, Massachusetts General Hospital/Harvard Medical School, Boston, MA.)*

- Melasma (Figure 3-17): skin condition characterized by hyper-pigmentation. Often associated with sun exposure plus oral contraceptive, other hormone use, or pregnancy (facial "mask of pregnancy"). Genetic and racial factors also may predispose to melasma. Melanin may be deposited in the basal and suprabasal layers or may be found in melanophages in the dermis. Both numbers and activity of melanocytes increased in melasma.

- Other conditions associated with hyperpigmentation:
  - Addison's disease: endocrine disorder characterized by brown hyperpigmentation of skin.
  - Pellagra: nutritional disorder (niacin deficiency) resulting in hyperpigmentation, especially prominent around the neck.
  - Incontinentia pigmenti: developmental disorder characterized by whorls of hyperpigmented patches.
  - Ochronosis: metabolic disorder characterized by blue-gray hyperpigmentation of sclera, pinnae, tip of the nose, and over extensor tendons of hand and fingernails.
  - Malignant disorders such as metastatic melanoma can cause hyperpigmentation of skin.
  - Chemically induced disorders can cause a wide variety of color changes in skin: clofazimine (red), mepacrine (yellow), antimalarial agents, gold, and amiodarone (slate gray), minocycline (blue-black skin and gum changes), and cyclophosphamide (brown to black pigmentation of nails and teeth).

■ Appearance
- Patches of increased pigmentation on any area of body
- If due to melasma: patches of hyperpigmentation, usually on malar, mandibular, or central areas of face

■ Diagnosis
- Patches of postinflammatory hyperpigmentation not diagnostic; merely "footprints" left behind inflammation
- Wood's lamp examination: enhancement of pigmentation if pigment in epidermis; no enhancement if pigmentation in dermis

■ Treatment
- Hyperpigmentation after inflammatory acne lesions: patient should be reassured that the condition will gradually resolve if area not further irritated.
- Skin bleaching creams containing hydroquinone sometimes helpful in treatment of small areas of skin hyperpigmentation if not irritating to skin. ***Caution:* Prior to using such creams on face, test dose should be applied overnight to antecubital fossae to make sure irritation does not occur. Despite negative test result, irritation could still occur; if so, cream should be discontinued. Irritation promotes further hyperpigmentation.**
- Protection against sunlight important in preventing further changes in pigmentation. Sunscreens used should protect against both UVA and UVB. Azelaic acid, retinoids, or bleaching agents containing hydroquinone may be useful in reducing hyperpigmentation from epidermal pigment.

DISORDERS INVOLVING THE BASEMENT MEMBRANE

Pemphigus (Figure 3-18)

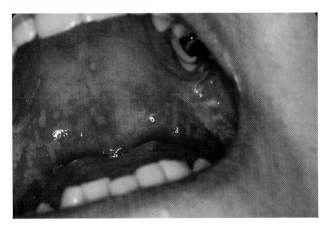

Figure 3-18 • Pemphigus. *(Image courtesy of Dr. Howard Baden, Massachusetts General Hospital/Harvard Medical School, Boston, MA.)*

■ **Definition**
- Autoimmune disease characterized by fragile, flaccid blisters in skin that break easily and form large, painful erosions on skin and mucous membranes
- Pemphigus vulgaris: fragile blisters on skin and mucous membranes
- Pemphigus foliaceous: fragile blisters, rupturing easily, scaling skin surface
- Paraneoplastic pemphigus: blisters, erosions, prominent mucous membrane erosions

■ **Etiology**
- Precipitating causes of pemphigus vulgaris and pemphigus foliaceous unknown.
- Pemphigus foliaceous: Endemic form occurs in Brazil, where distribution of disease correlates with habitat of the black (biting) fly, *Simulium pruinosum*.
- Paraneoplastic pemphigus: associated with underlying neoplasms, often occult. In cases where the underlying neoplasm is successfully treated, paraneoplastic pemphigus will greatly improve or resolve.

■ **Appearance**

- Lesions often first appear on roof of mouth and spread to skin and intertriginous areas (axilla, groin, buttock crease).
- Often involvement of proximal esophagus, causing pain on swallowing.
- Upper epidermis easily peels from underlying basal layer of cells (called Nikolsky's sign); can be tested by pressing on blister to see if blister extends.

■ **Diagnosis**

- Biopsy:
  - Pemphigus vulgaris: IgG autoantibodies against cell surface of keratinocytes responsible for detachment of cells. Histopathology: suprabasalar acantholysis (separation of epidermis from basal cell layer). Cells left behind in basal cell layer resemble "row of tombstones."
  - Pemphigus foliaceous: blister occurs in granular layer instead of above the basal layer. Granular layer is higher in the skin layers; therefore, blister has less "roof" to it, and is fragile, rupturing easily.
  - In paraneoplastic pemphigus, there is suprabasalar acantholysis as in pemphigus vulgaris but there is also substantial inflammatory cell infiltrate, unlike pemphigus vulgaris.
- Blood test for circulating antibodies: Most patients have circulating IgG antibodies that bind to the keratinocyte surface; the titer of these antibodies usually correlates with the severity of the disease.

■ **Treatment**

- Systemic therapy with steroids or other immunosuppressives (cyclophosphamide or azathioprine). Before oral corticosteroids were available, disease had 100% mortality within 5 years. Risk for infection nevertheless remains, and most affected patients require lifelong therapy.

Bullous Pemphigoid (Figure 3-19)

■ **Definition**

- Acquired autoimmune blistering disease that affects the skin

■ **Etiology**

- Unknown

■ **Appearance**

- Patients with bullous pemphigoid are usually elderly and have tense blisters on an erythematous base or on normal-appearing skin.

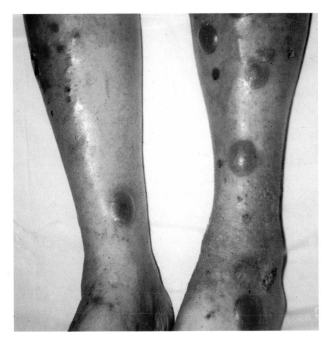

Figure 3-19 • Bullous pemphigoid. *(Image courtesy of Dr. Howard Baden, Massachusetts General Hospital/Harvard Medical School, Boston, MA.)*

- Blisters are usually found on lower trunk, extremities, groin, and axillae.
- Itching may be severe.
- Mucosal involvement transient; not predominant feature.
- Nikolsky's phenomenon absent.

■ Diagnosis

- Biopsy: Histopathologic evaluation of biopsy specimen shows blister formation in lamina lucida, part of basement membrane.
- Blood test for circulating antibodies: Patients have circulating IgG antibodies against two antigens that are part of hemidesmosomes that adhere basal cell to basement membrane.

■ Treatment

- Mild localized disease can be treated with topical steroids. Patients with more extensive disease may require oral steroids.
- To avoid steroid use in elderly, combination of tetracycline (2 g per day) and niacinamide (1.5 g per day) sometimes used.
- Mycophenolate mofetil, an immunosuppressive agent, may also be useful.

Lichen Planus

■ Definition

- Inflammatory disorder with bandlike lymphocytic infiltrate in upper dermis, resulting in degeneration of basal layer of skin

■ Etiology

- No known cause

■ Appearance

- Lesions of lichen planus are flat-topped, violaceous, polygonal-shaped papules, usually on the flexor surface of the wrist and arms; sometimes on the legs or trunk.
- Fine scale and delicate white lines (Wickham's striae) often found on papules, and lacy white lesions often found on buccal mucosa, gingiva, and underside of tongue.
- Lesions are often itchy.
- As in psoriasis, Koebner's phenomenon is present, wherein trauma to normal skin causes lesions of lichen planus to arise in the traumatized areas.

■ Diagnosis

- Biopsy: Histology shows dense bandlike infiltrates of T-lymphocytes and histiocytes in upper dermis that obscure basement membrane area and are associated with damage to basal layer of skin, suggesting T cell-mediated attack against antigens in basal layer. Necrotic keratinocytes from basal layer drop down into papillary dermis, where they are called colloid bodies. In some cases of lichen planus, clefts at the dermoepidermal junction result in vesicle formation.

■ Treatment

- Topical corticosteroids or PUVA

DISORDERS OF THE DERMIS

Ehlers-Danlos Syndrome (Figure 3-20)

■ Definition

- Group of inherited disorders of collagen metabolism, characterized by tissue fragility

■ Etiology

- Group of inherited disorders or autoimmune dysfunction that impair balance of synthesis and degradation of collagen in the dermis

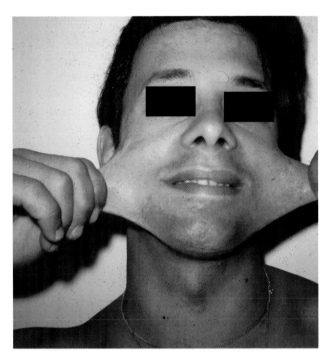

Figure 3-20 • Ehlers-Danlos syndrome. *(Image courtesy of Dr. Howard Baden, Massachusetts General Hospital/Harvard Medical School, Boston, MA.)*

■ **Appearance**
- Skin fragility and hyperextensibility, as well as loose jointedness
- May develop rupture of the aorta or other arterial blood vessels

■ **Diagnosis**
- Clinical appearance, genetic studies, biopsy. ***Caution:*** **Skin does not heal well after surgery, may have large, "fish-mouth" scars.**

■ **Treatment**
- None available

Epidermolysis Bullosa (Figure 3-21)

■ **Definition**
- Genetic disorders characterized by blisters and varying degrees of scarring

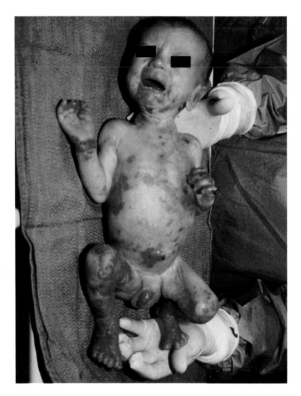

Figure 3-21 • Epidermolysis bullosa. *(Image courtesy of Dr. Howard Baden, Massachusetts General Hospital/Harvard Medical School, Boston, MA.)*

■ Etiology/Pathophysiology

- Genetic: Epidermis is anchored to dermis via an "anchoring complex" that includes "anchoring filaments" (laminin 5) that connect basal cells to the basement membrane and "anchoring fibrils" (collagen type VII) that anchor the basement membrane to the dermis. Defects in these or other components of the anchoring complex can result in loss of epidermal anchor to the dermis and in blister formation.

- There are dominant and recessive inheritance patterns and different mutations resulting in different clinical presentations with different degrees of severity and scarring.
  - Epidermolysis bullosa simplex: defects in keratins 5 or 14 (found in basal cells); blistering; normally no scarring
  - Junctional epidermolysis bullosa: defects in hemidesmosomes or anchoring filaments; may be scarring or no scarring
  - Dystrophic epidermolysis bullosa: defects in anchoring fibrils; servere scarring in recessive type

- Autoimmune: Epidermolysis bullosa can also occur as a result from autoimmunity to type VII collagen (epidermolysis bullosa acquisita).

■ **Appearance**

- In Hallopeau-Siemens type of recessive dystrophic epidermolysis bullosa, anchoring fibrils are absent; blistering and mutilating scarring result; aggressive squamous cell carcinomas may develop in eroded and scarred areas of skin.
- Less severe form (blister formation occurring higher in the skin): epidermolysis bullosa simplex (blisters develop within epidermis), no scarring.
- In junctional epidermolysis bullosa, blisters develop between the basal layer of cells and the basal lamina of the basement membrane.
- Regardless of the type of epidermolysis bullosa, blistering is a common feature.

■ **Diagnosis**

- Biopsy: Level of blister formation and clinical appearance will help distinguish type.

■ **Treatment**

- Monitor for development of squamous cell carcinoma.
- Monitor for superimposed infection: treat with antibiotics (topical or oral) as necessary.
- Protection of skin from trauma.

Keloid Scars and Hypertrophic Scars

■ **Definition**

- Keloid scars: large scars that overgrow the line of injury or surgery, forming irregular, bulbous borders. Hypertrophic scars: similar appearance, but follow line of injury or surgery.

■ **Etiology**

- Keloid scars and hypertrophic scars caused by increased rate of synthesis of collagen in dermis, usually following injury or surgical procedure to area.
- Reason for excessive synthesis of collagen not understood, but genetic component appears to be involved.
- Dark-skinned individuals appear to have increased risk for developing keloid scars.

■ **Appearance/Clinical**

- Keloid scars and hypertrophic scars often itch; keloids can be painful. Surgical excision of keloid can result in recurrence of larger scar.

■ Diagnosis
- Clinical appearance of keloid scar or hypertrophic scar usually sufficient for diagnosis.
- Biopsy of either type of scar will show thick, eosinophilic bands of collagen and whorls of fibroblasts and fibrous tissue in haphazard arrangement, resulting in thickened dermis.

■ Treatment
- Keloid scars and hypertrophic scars can be treated with intralesional steroids, injections once a month until growth stops and flattening of scar occurs.
- Large keloids can be treated with surgical or laser excision followed by intralesional steroids to surgical site, given once a month for several months.

Scleroderma (Figure 3-22)

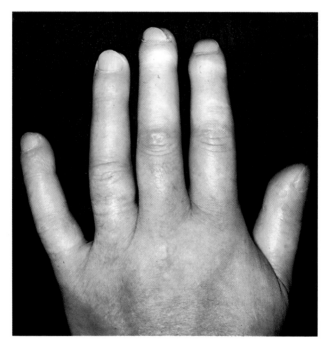

Figure 3-22 • Scleroderma. *(Image courtesy of Dr. Howard Baden, Massachusetts General Hospital/Harvard Medical School, Boston, MA.)*

See also the section on Scleroderma in Chapter 6.

■ **Definition**

• Disorder of excess collagen production

■ **Etiology/Pathophysiology**

• Scleroderma is autoimmune disease of unknown etiology.
• Has been speculated that infection, hereditary factors, or chemical substances in environment may play role in etiology.
• Excess collagen deposited in dermis, obliterating blood vessels; overlying skin becomes atrophic.

■ **Appearance/Clinical Presentation**

• Systemic disease can be either limited or diffuse.
• Onset of systemic scleroderma usually manifested first in hands and feet, where diffuse swelling, blanching, or other color changes, and tingling or numbness (Raynaud's phenomenon) occur, especially in response to cold.
• Skin on hands, feet, and other parts of body become thickened and immobile.
• Skin feels thick and tight.
• Skin of fingers becomes bound down to underlying structures (sclerodactyly) and loses flexibility.
• Fingers tapered; contractures of hands; skin calcifications.
• Facial skin tightens, obliterating wrinkles except around the mouth, where they are prominent.
• Skin over nose becomes tight, resulting in "beaklike" appearance.
• Lines of normal facial expression lost; facial telangiectasias prominent.
• The mouth appears smaller; lips are thin.
• Internal organs affected.
• Fibrosis and vascular injury occurs, most commonly in heart, resulting in heart blocks and arrhythmias.
• Pulmonary fibrosis and pulmonary arterial hypertension.
• Kidney sclerosis resulting in renal crisis.
• Esophageal dysmotility, dyspepsia, constipation.
• Scleroderma occurs also in localized forms.
  - Morphea: white or yellowish plaques of thickened skin
  - Linear scleroderma (Figure 3-23): thickened skin and atrophy in a linear distribution

■ **Diagnosis**

• Diagnosis of scleroderma depends on clinical picture of symmetric thickening as well as tightening and induration of skin.
• May be pitting scars or loss of substance from finger pad.
• Bibasilar pulmonary fibrosis may be present.
• Antinuclear antibodies likely to be present, with anticentromere pattern common in patients with limited disease.

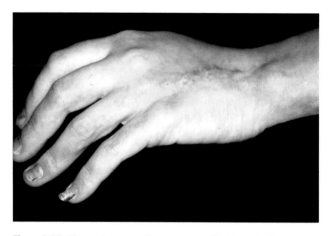

Figure 3-23 • Linear scleroderma. *(Image courtesy of Dr. Howard Baden, Massachusetts General Hospital/Harvard Medical School, Boston, MA.)*

- In patients with diffuse disease, antibodies to SCL-70 (topoi-somerase I) common.
- Biopsy: thinned epidermis and thickened collagen bundles in dermis, replacing adnexal structures.

■ Treatment

- Cases of scleroderma should be referred to expert for management.
- No satisfactory treatment, but several medications useful in relieving some symptoms. Calcium channel blockers help relieve symptoms of Raynaud's phenomenon. D-Penicillamine (inhibits cross-linkage of collagen) gives some relief to inflexibility of skin and accumulation of collagen. Oral corticosteroids sometimes helpful but may contribute to renal crisis. Other treatments under investigation include cyclosporine, interferon-gamma, and extra-corporeal photochemotherapy.

Granuloma Annulare (Figure 3-24)

■ Definition

- Condition of unknown origin characterized by pink or flesh-colored papules in annular configuration(s)
- Lesions usually asymptomatic; can appear on any part of the body (hands, feet most commonly affected)

■ Etiology/Pathophysiology

- Cause unknown
- Has been reported in association with diabetes, but little sup-port for a true relationship

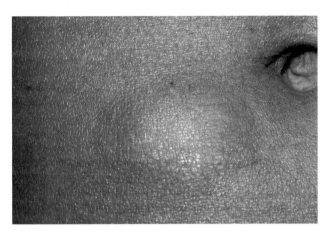

Figure 3-24 • Granuloma annulare. *(Image courtesy of Dr. Howard Baden, Massachusetts General Hospital/Harvard Medical School, Boston, MA.)*

■ **Appearance**
- May be mistaken for ringworm (tinea corporis) but differs in that no scale is present in granuloma annulare since, unlike ringworm, it is a lesion arising from the dermis instead of from the epidermis.

■ **Diagnosis**
- Clinical appearance plus biopsy will confirm the diagnosis.
- Biopsy: inflammation with areas of degenerative collagen (as opposed to scleroderma, which is associated with inflammation and increased collagen deposition).

■ **Treatment**
- Spontaneous resolution of lesions sometimes occurs.
- Injection of triamcinolone or cryotherapy can be helpful.
- For widespread granuloma annulare: reports of some success with dapsone or PUVA therapy.

DISORDERS OF THE SUBCUTANEOUS FAT

Panniculitis

■ **Definition**
- Inflammatory disorders of the subcutaneous fat
  - Lobular panniculitis: inflammation in fat lobules
  - Septal panniculitis: inflammation in fibrous septa surrounding the lobules

■ **Etiology**

- Often unknown
- Infection
- Autoimmune disorders

■ **Appearance**

- Erythematous or violaceous nodules, often on the lower extremities.
- Nodules sometimes ulcerate.

■ **Diagnosis**

- Biopsy

■ **Treatment**

- Anti-inflammatory medication, antibiotics as necessary

Erythema Nodosum

■ **Definition**

- Septal panniculitis with inflammatory cells invading the septa and adjacent fat cells

■ **Etiology**

- Hypersensitivity reaction, often to medications or wide variety of bacterial, viral, or fungal diseases.
- More common in females.
- Reactive phenomena set off by number of causes, including medications, infection (tuberculosis, histoplasmosis, sarcoidosis), inflammatory bowel disease.
- Oral contraceptives sometimes precipitate erythema nodosum.
- Can be associated with malignant disease such as Hodgkin's disease or leukemia and with conditions such as Crohn's disease, hepatitis, or tuberculosis.
- Often no cause found.

■ **Appearance**

- Painful and erythematous nodules on the anterior lower legs

■ **Diagnosis**

- Biopsy
- Chest x-ray if sarcoid, tuberculosis, or histoplasmosis suspected (erythema nodosum and shortness of breath)

■ **Treatment**

- Treat underlying disease.
- Aspirin or other nonsteroidal anti-inflammatory medications, potassium iodide (400–900 mg daily or 2–10 drops of a saturated

solution tid), or injection of nodules with triamcinolone can be helpful in relieving symptoms.

Erythema Induratum

■ **Definition**
- Nodular panniculitis
- Erythema induratum, also called Bazin's disease.

■ **Etiology**
- Thought to be caused by vascular hypersensitivity reaction, in the past often associated with tuberculosis
- Likely caused by an immune complex-mediated vascular injury

■ **Appearance**
- Usually in females with tender, erythematous nodules or plaques on the lower legs that become blue-red and ulcerate, leaving scars

■ **Diagnosis**
- Biopsy: Histologically there are tuberculoid granulomas, caseating necrosis in the fat lobules, and vasculitis in medium-sized vessels and venules in the fibrous septa. Epitheloid cells surround areas of necrosis, as well as lymphocytes, foreign-body giant cells, polymorphonuclear leukocytes, and plasma cells.
- Tuberculin skin test should be performed to rule out tuberculosis prior to treatment with systemic steroids.

■ **Treatment**
- Nonsteroidal anti-inflammatory medications or tetracycline may also be helpful.

DISORDERS OF THE VASCULATURE

Stasis Dermatitis (Figure 3-25)

■ **Definition**
- Chronic condition characterized by eczematous changes of skin of lower legs

■ **Etiology/Pathophysiology**
- Underlying problem is venous insufficiency and calf muscle pump dysfunction. Legs swell, causing skin stretching and damage. Inflammation results, and over time dermal fibrosis and sclerosis occur.

■ **Appearance**
- Skin changes can include edema, erythema, scaling, weeping, and petechiae, and secondary infection can occur and progress into cellulitis.

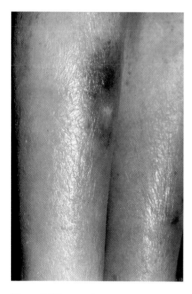

Figure 3-25 • Statis dermatitis. *(Image courtesy of Dr. Howard Baden, Massachusetts General Hospital/Harvard Medical School, Boston, MA.)*

- Histologically: thick-walled capillaries in fibrotic dermis, extravasated erythrocytes (blood cells outside of the vessels), spongiosis of epidermis and fibrin thrombi in vascular lumina.

■ **Diagnosis**
- Clinical appearance usually sufficient for diagnosis.
- Biopsy can confirm diagnosis if in doubt.

■ **Treatment**
- Leg elevation, support hose.
- Application of mild topical corticosteroids to reduce inflammation.
- Increase in erythema and tenderness should suggest possible superimposed infection.
- Infection can usually be treated with cephalosporins, erythromycin, or penicillin.

Vasculitis (Figure 3-26)

■ **Definition**
- Inflammation and necrosis of blood vessel walls.
- Some types of vasculitis affect small vessels, others affect large vessels, and still others affect both. Some affect arteries, others affect veins.

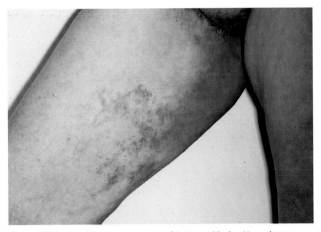

Figure 3-26 • Vasculitis. *(Image courtesy of Dr. Howard Baden, Massachusetts General Hospital/Harvard Medical School, Boston, MA.)*

■ **Etiology**
- Often unknown
- Infection, autoimmune diseases
- Allergic cutaneous vasculitis can occur secondary to drugs
- Thiazides sometimes cause such reactions
- Temporal arteritis, polyarteritis nodosa, Wegener's granulomatosis, and Churg-Strauss syndrome are examples of other disorders with vasculitis.

■ **Appearance**
- Effects may be manifested only in the skin or may be part of widespread systemic involvement.

■ **Diagnosis**
- Biopsy important in determining whether vasculitis present and what types of vessels involved

■ **Treatment**
- Treatment of underlying disorder

DISORDERS OF THE EPIDERMIS, DERMIS, AND VASCULATURE

Rosacea (Figure 3-27)

■ **Definition**
- Common, chronic inflammatory condition, more frequently found in fair-skinned individuals; affects epidermis, dermis, and vasculature

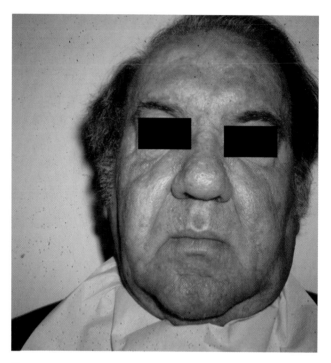

Figure 3-27 • Rosacea. *(Image courtesy of Dr. Howard Baden, Massachusetts General Hospital/Harvard Medical School, Boston, MA.)*

■ **Etiology**
- Cause unknown.
- May involve sensitivity to *Demodex folliculorum* mites, normally found in follicles of face.
- Foods or activities that stimulate flushing can exacerbate rosacea; elastotic changes from sun damage noted in biopsy samples of rosacea prompt theory that ultraviolet damage has caused loss of vascular integrity, resulting in vasodilation, development of telangiectasia, and inflammation.

■ **Appearance**
- Facial erythema, telangiectasias, inflammatory papules and pustules, and sometimes tissue hyperplasia from granulomatous changes in dermis, especially on nose where rhinophyma (bulbous growths) may occur.
- Rhinophyma occurs more frequently in males, unusual in females.

- Facial flushing can often occur and persist. Rosacea primarily affects nose, malar area, forehead, and chin. Can also be eye involvement resulting in conjunctivitis, blepharitis, and keratitis.

■ **Diagnosis**
- Diagnosis usually made on clinical presentation alone.
- Biopsy: Telangiectasia, noncaseating epithelioid granulomas around follicles, and perivascular infiltrates of lymphocytes and histiocytes; also sebaceous hyperplasia and dermal fibrosis in areas of rhinophyma.

■ **Treatment**
- Topical metronidazole, oral antibiotics such as tetracycline, or topical antibiotics such as clindamycin or erythromycin
- Sunscreen use important

Psoriasis

- Psoriasis is another example of disorder that affects epidermis, dermis, and vasculature.
- There are tortuous vessels in the papillary (upper) dermis and hyperkeratosis and acanthosis of the epidermis. Psoriasis was discussed earlier in this chapter.

Skin Conditions Caused by the External Environment

- Location and distribution of skin changes can often point to the cause.
- History of recent or concurrent viral illness may give valuable clues.
- New medication or new sensitivity to an old medication may have precipitated a skin eruption.

CONTACT DERMATITIS

- Most people develop irritant contact dermatitis immediately following contact with an irritating substance (e.g., lye or ammonia).
- Contact with poison ivy causes allergic contact dermatitis (Figure 4-1, allergic contact dermatitis to red dye in tattoo) in some but not in others, depending on whether sensitization of the individual has previously occurred.
- Allergic contact dermatitis is an immunologic reaction involving T-cell pathways; clinical manifestations are delayed in onset.

Poison Ivy

■ Definition

- Contact with poison ivy usually results in allergic contact dermatitis.

■ Etiology

- The allergen is oil found on leaves of the poison ivy plant.
- Allergic contact dermatitis is an example of delayed-hypersensitivity, cell-mediated immune disease (type IV).
- With the help of Langerhans' cells in skin, antigen is processed and presented to the T cell, which activates T cells that proliferate and secrete lymphokines and inflammatory cytokines. Skin responds with erythema and vesicle formation; memory T cells are formed that allow quicker reaction to the antigen if it invades on another occasion.
- Rash of poison ivy can also be acquired in an airborne manner from smoke of burning poison ivy plants. In such cases, eruption appears on the face and other exposed parts.

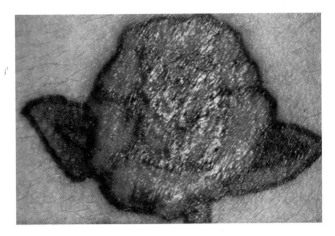

Figure 4-1 • Contact dermatitis (to red in tattoo). *(Image courtesy of Dr. Howard Baden, Massachusetts General Hospital/Harvard Medical School, Boston, MA.)*

■ **Appearance**
• Vesicles, plaques, erythema, exudates, crust

■ **Diagnosis**
• Can usually be diagnosed by clinical appearance and history

■ **Treatment**
• Tapering dose of oral corticosteroids or application of topical corticosteroids for localized patches.
• Oral antihistamines help relieve intense itching accompanying skin eruption.
• For localized patches of poison ivy dermatitis, strong topical corticosteroids may be helpful.
• Wash clothes, gloves, or other objects that have come in contact with poison ivy.
• Bathe pets that have come in contact with poison ivy plants. Plant oil can adhere to animal fur.

Diaper Rash

■ **Definition**
• Example of irritant contact dermatitis

■ **Etiology**
• Reaction of baby's skin to ammonia in urine; sometimes secondary infection from feces.

- *Note:* Many other factors in the environment can cause irritant or allergic contact dermatitis; among the most common are perfume, nickel (jewelry, buckles), shoe leather, bulb plants, clothing containing formaldehyde, and elastic. The area of dermatitis will usually map to the area that has come in contact with an irritating or allergenic substance.

■ **Appearance**
- Papules, plaques, erythema, vesicles, erosion

■ **Diagnosis**
- Diagnosed from clinical appearance.
- Culture may be helpful if secondary infection suspected.

■ **Treatment**
- Avoidance of irritant or allergen.
- Prevention of diaper rash involves changing diapers often, using super-absorbable diapers, and applying zinc oxide ointment or petrolatum to diaper area after cleansing.
- Application of topical corticosteroid can be helpful in treatment of irritant contact dermatitis. Oral corticosteroids and oral antihistamines can be helpful in treatment of allergic contact dermatitis.
- *Note:* Only class 6 (see Appendix B) corticosteroids should be used on the face, groin, or axilla, where skin is thin and absorption greater than on other parts of the body. Other classes can be used on other parts of the body as appropriate, but class 1 corticosteroids should not be used for more than 2 weeks at a time (then a 2-week "holiday" with use of a milder corticosteroid should take place before restarting the class 1 corticosteroid). For maximum penetration of corticosteroid in persistent areas, the corticosteroid, if class 2 to 6, can be used under occlusion, but class 1 corticosteroids should not be occluded. Inappropriate use of corticosteroids can result in thinning of skin, development of telangiectasia, and development of striae ("stretch marks"). Occlusion enhances skin penetration of corticosteroid but also provides good environment for bacterial overgrowth. Systemic absorption is rare but can occur with high-potency topical corticosteroids.

Contact Urticaria

■ **Definition**
- Immediate development of urticaria (hives) or angioedema
- IgE-mediated, immediate-hypersensitivity response
- Can occasionally result in anaphylactic reaction

■ **Etiology**
- Latex allergy is an example of allergy that can result in contact urticaria.

■ **Appearance**
- Swelling of face, lips, mucosa upon contact with an irritating or sensitizing substance

■ **Diagnosis**
- Clinical appearance

■ **Treatment**
- Patient to ER.
- Avoidance of latex products crucial for persons with latex allergy.
- Contact with latex can result in medical emergency with need for immediate treatment with antihistamines, epinephrine, and corticosteroids.

BURNS

- Result of thermal or chemical insult from the environment to skin.
- Severe burns best managed in burn unit of a hospital.
- Minor burns can usually be managed with topical silver sulfadiazine (Silvadene) and careful wound care.
- Make certain that patient has had recent tetanus shot; monitor for superimposed infection.
- Chemical burns must be flushed well with normal saline to remove residual chemical.

MECHANICAL IRRITATION OF THE SKIN

- Mechanical irritation of skin can result in abrasion, laceration, bullae, erosion, ulceration, corns and calluses, and other problems.

Corns

■ **Definition**
- Hyperkeratotic, often annular plaques and papules on feet

■ **Etiology**
- Occur as a result of friction and pressure caused by shoes and body weight

■ **Appearance**

• May be soft, hard, vascular, or neurovascular; can be very painful
• Lack of thrombosed capillaries characteristic of warts

■ **Diagnosis**

• Diagnosis by clinical appearance

■ **Treatment**

• Salicylic acid plasters followed by paring are effective treatment for corns.
• Avoid tight-fitting shoes to prevent recurrence.

Ingrown Toenails

■ **Definition**

• Ingrown toenails (onychocryptosis)

■ **Etiology**

• Can result from incorrect nail trimming, from shoes that bind, or from other activities that put stress on growing nail.
• Secondary bacterial infection can occur that causes discomfort and results in cellulitis or other problems.

■ **Treatment**

• Treatment of bacterial infection with antibiotics necessary; partial or total nail avulsion may be helpful.
• Partial or total nail avulsion sometimes followed by partial or total matrix destruction to prevent regrowth of portion of nail that is troublesome.

SOLAR-INDUCED DISORDERS

Actinic Keratoses (Figure 4-2)

■ **Definition**

• Precancerous lesions found in sun-exposed areas.
• Some of these lesions may change over time into squamous cell carcinoma.

■ **Etiology**

• Induced by sun exposure
• Occur in largest numbers in fair-skinned individuals that live in or travel to sunny climates

■ **Appearance**

• Erythematous papules or macules with scale
• Can often be felt as tiny spots that feel rough like sandpaper, even if too small to be seen

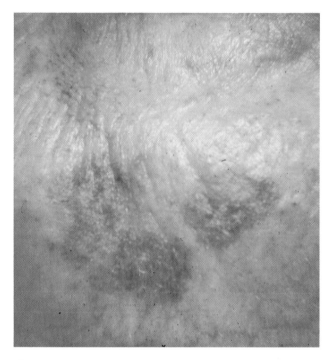

Figure 4-2 • Actinic keratoses. *(Image courtesy of Dr. Howard Baden, Massachusetts General Hospital/Harvard Medical School, Boston, MA.)*

■ **Diagnosis**
- Diagnosis usually made from clinical appearance.
- Biopsy if in doubt.

■ **Treatment**
- Early treatment important.
- Treatment with liquid nitrogen, curettage, excision, or topical 5-fluorouracil.
- Check patient every 6 to 12 months and counsel on importance of sun protection.

Solar Lentigines

■ **Definition**
- Sun stimulates melanocytes to proliferate, resulting in dark brown-black color of lentigines (lentigo, singular).

■ **Etiology**
- Induced by sun exposure

■ **Appearance**
- Dark macules or patches often found on backs of hands and on face

■ **Diagnosis**
- Biopsy should be performed on lentigines that develop black or multicolored pigmentation to rule out lentigo maligna or melanoma *in situ*.

■ **Treatment**
- No treatment necessary for lentigines

Phototoxic, Photoallergic Reactions (Figure 4-3)

■ **Definition**
- Phototoxic or photoallergic reaction, resulting in rash or burn

■ **Etiology**
- Phototoxic reaction: sun exposure (UV radiation), combined with orally ingested or topically applied phototoxic substance (e.g., thiazides and furocoumarins)
  - *Note:* **Furocoumarins include psoralens, fragrances, and some plants and vegetables (lime, celery, carrots, figs, parsley, parsnips).**
  - Phototoxic reaction involves nonimmunologic mechanisms
  - *Note:* **Because exposure to sun can be beneficial in treatment of psoriasis, psoralens are used orally or topically in PUVA treatment of this disease.**
- Photoallergic reaction: involves delayed sensitivity to photosensitizing agent and exposure to ultraviolet radiation
  - Only persons previously sensitized to particular substance will be affected.
  - Musk ambrette, contained in some fragrances, and Parsol, ingredient found in some sunscreens, are examples of potential photoallergens.

■ **Appearance**
- Phototoxic: Erythema (like sunburn); affected skin stings and burns.
- Photoallergic: Erythema (like sunburn); affected skin itches.

■ **Treatment**
- Treatment with topical corticosteroids helpful in reducing erythema.
- Oral antihistamines to reduce itching.

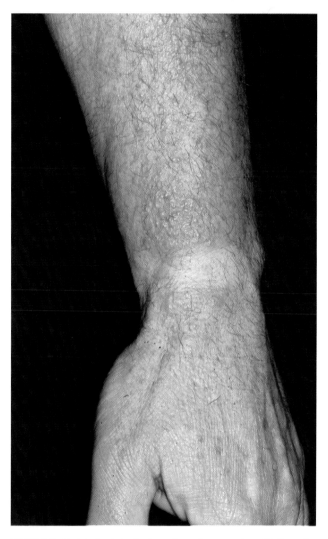

Figure 4-3 • Phototoxic, photoallergic reactions. *(Image courtesy of Dr. Howard Baden, Massachusetts General Hospital/Harvard Medical School, Boston, MA.)*

- *Note:* Avoid topical antihistamines. They can irritate skin.
- Prevention of reactions by avoidance of sun, use of sunscreens. Avoidance of precipitating substance.

Photoaging

- Sun not only increases likelihood that skin cancer will develop, but also causes skin wrinkling, sagging, and color changes associated with aging.
- Photoaging can be diminished by protection from the sun (use of sunscreens and protective clothing).
- Sun protection should start early: sun damage is cumulative, and effects of sun exposure in childhood and the teen years will be reaped later in life.

5 Skin Infections and Infestations

FUNGAL INFECTIONS OF SKIN

Most fungi that infect the stratum corneum of skin are called dermatophytes and fall within three main genera: *Epidermophyton*, *Microsporum*, and *Trichophyton*. Most fungi that infect hair are within the *Microsporum* and *Trichophyton* genera. Piedra is a superficial mycosis of the hair shaft. There are two varieties of piedra: black piedra (Figure 5-1), caused by *Piedraia hortae*, and white piedra, caused by *Trichosporon beigelii*. Tinea nigra is a superficial infection of the epidermis caused by *Phaeoannellomyces werneckii* (*Exophiala werneckii*). There are also deep fungal infections of skin that are uncommon except in immunocompromised patients.

The types of superficial fungal infections are outlined in Table 5-1.

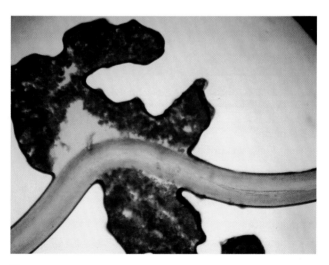

Figure 5-1 • Black piedra. *(Image courtesy of Dr. Howard Baden, Massachusetts General Hospital/Harvard Medical School, Boston, MA.)*

■ TABLE 5-1 Fungal Infections

Tinea capitis	Hair
Onychomycosis	Nails
Tinea manus	Hands
Tinea pedis	Feet
Tinea cruris	Groin
Tinea facei	Face other than beard area
Tinea barbae	Beard area of face
Tinea corporis	Other areas of skin

Tinea Corporis (Figure 5-2)

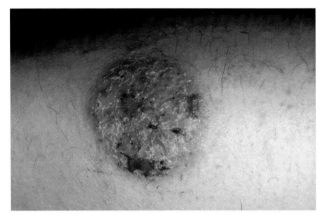

Figure 5-2 • Tinea corporis. *(Image courtesy of Dr. Howard Baden, Massachusetts General Hospital/Harvard Medical School, Boston, MA.)*

■ Definition
- Fungal infection involving trunk or extremities

■ Etiology
- Dermatophytes, usually within the genera of *Epidermophyton*, *Microsporum*, and *Trichophyton*

■ Appearance
- Plaques with erythema and scale, central clearing

■ Diagnosis
- Skin scraping and hyphae seen under microscope

■ Treatment
- Topical antifungal such as ketoconazole (Nizoral) usually is sufficient; oral antifungal may be used in severe cases.

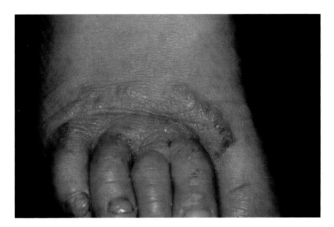

Figure 5-3 • Tinea pedis. *(Image courtesy of Dr. Howard Baden, Massachusetts General Hospital/Harvard Medical School, Boston, MA.)*

■ Comment

Fungal infections usually appear as plaques with erythema and scale and are often in an annular configuration with central clearing (Figures 5-3 and 5-4). Fungi and yeast can be identified by their

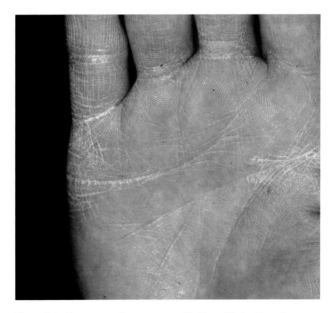

Figure 5-4 • Tinea manus. *(Image courtesy of Dr. Howard Baden, Massachusetts General Hospital/Harvard Medical School, Boston, MA.)*

morphology in tissue (skin scrapings), by growth morphology on Sabouraud's agar and other special media, and by responsiveness to certain laboratory tests. In practice, observing hyphae in skin scrapings under the microscope or receiving positive culture results is usually sufficient for treatment. Specific typing is not usually necessary except in persistent or otherwise unusual cases.

Topical antifungals are usually sufficient for treating infections with limited distribution. For more widespread involvement or for infection of hair or nails, oral antifungals may be necessary. If oral antifungals are used, liver functions should be monitored before and during treatment.

YEAST INFECTIONS OF SKIN

Yeast can also infect skin. *Candida albicans* is pathogenic for skin if it gains a foothold. Some of the normally saphrophytic species of *Candida* can also cause infection if overgrowth occurs because of erosion, occlusion, and other factors that promote yeast growth.

Pityriasis Versicolor

■ **Definition**
- Pityriasis versicolor (tinea versicolor): superficial fungal infection

■ **Etiology**
- Yeast: *Malassezia furfur*
- Most cases occur in moist, warm climates

■ **Appearance**
- Hypopigmentation or hyperpigmentation, salmon-colored macules and patches with scale
- Most often found on the upper back and upper chest
- Occasionally pruritic (itchy), otherwise asymptomatic

■ **Diagnosis**
- Scraping and examination with KOH preparation: "spaghetti and meatballs" appearance of short hyphae and round yeast forms

■ **Treatment**
- 2.5% selenium sulfide lotion (Selsun lotion), or shampoo containing zinc pyrithione (Zincon shampoo) applied for 5 to 10 minutes prior to showering every day for 2 weeks
- Itraconazole 200 or 400 mg orally once or twice a month useful prophylactically

Intertrigo (Figure 5-5)

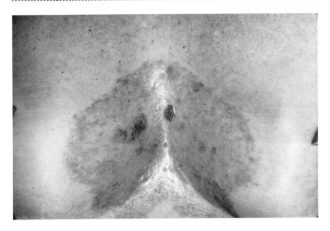

Figure 5-5 • Intertrigo. *(Image courtesy of Dr. Howard Baden, Massachusetts General Hospital/Harvard Medical School, Boston, MA.)*

■ **Definition**
- Irritation of intertriginous areas (buttock creases, groin, between fingers and toes, under breasts)

■ **Etiology**
- Yeast likes to grow in moist, warm intertriginous areas, especially when the skin is chapped or macerated for any reason.
- Intertrigo can also be caused by bacterial infection, especially if between the fingers and toes. *Corynebacterium* are often the bacterial agents involved.

■ **Appearance**
- Erythematous plaques and patches in intertriginous areas

■ **Diagnosis**
- Clinical appearance usually sufficient for diagnosis

■ **Treatment**
- Antifungal cream such as topical ketoconazole cream.
- Mild corticosteroid can be added if there is much irritation. ***Note:* Vytone cream, containing both hydrocortisone and iodoquinone (antifungal) is helpful.**

- If bacterial infection is suspected (between fingers and toes), use topical erythromycin ointment 2% bid.

Angular Cheilitis (Figure 5-6)

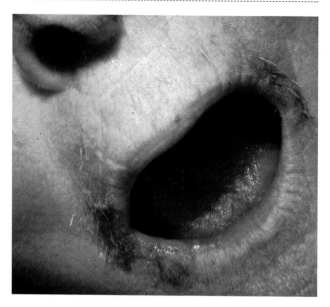

Figure 5-6 • Angular cheilitis. *(Image courtesy of Dr. Howard Baden, Massachusetts General Hospital/Harvard Medical School, Boston, MA.)*

■ **Definition**
- Inflammation of commissures of lips (sides of the mouth)

■ **Etiology**
- Irritation of skin folds can occur from drooling or lip licking.
- Yeast (*Candida*) superinfection can occur.

■ **Appearance**
- Cracks, fissures, and erythema of commissures of lips

■ **Diagnosis**
- Clinical appearance

■ **Treatment**
- Ketoconazole cream to affected areas bid

BACTERIAL INFECTIONS OF SKIN

Impetigo (Figure 5-7)

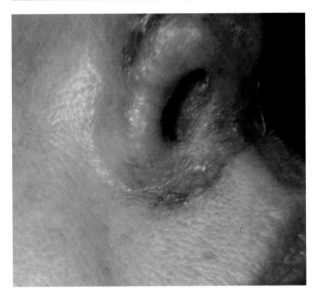

Figure 5-7 • Impetigo. *(Image courtesy of Dr. Howard Baden, Massachusetts General Hospital/Harvard Medical School, Boston, MA.)*

■ **Definition**
- Skin infection caused by *Staphylococcus* or *Streptococcus* organisms

■ **Etiology**
- Usually *Staphylococcus aureus* or *Streptococcus pyogenes*.
- A bullous form of impetigo, characterized by vesicles and bullae, can result from certain strains of *S. aureus* (including phage II, group 71, which produces a toxin causing separation in the granular layer of the epidermis).

■ **Appearance**
- Plaques and erosions, usually with yellowish crust
- Bullae, if bullous form

■ **Diagnosis**
- Infection is superficial in skin, and diagnosis of impetigo can usually be made on the basis of clinical appearance.

- Histopathologic examination shows vesicopustule formation just below the stratum corneum.

■ Treatment

- Impetigo is contagious and needs to be treated with antibiotics.
- Oral dicloxacillin (500 mg bid), erythromycin (500 mg bid), or a first-generation cephalosporin such as cephalexin (500 mg bid) will usually clear the lesions.
- If only a few lesions are present, topical mupiricin may be successful in clearing the problem.
- *Caution:* **Some strains of *S. pyogenes* that cause impetigo can cause poststreptococcal glomerulonephritis; early treatment is therefore important.**

Furuncles (Boils) and Carbuncles

■ Definition

- Furuncle (boil): deep inflammation and infection of the hair follicle; individual lesion with one follicular orifice
- Carbuncle: coalescing of infection from several adjacent follicles; several follicular orifices

■ Etiology

- Usually staphylococci

■ Appearance

- Furuncle: nodule with pustular formation and inflammation; most commonly on the legs, face, and groin
- Carbuncle: larger than furuncle, larger pustular component, often found on the posterior neck or buttocks

■ Diagnosis

- Culture may be helpful.

■ Treatment

- Incision, drainage, and oral antibiotics

Chancroid

■ Definition

- Sexually transmitted disease caused by contact with an infected partner

■ Etiology

- *Haemophilus ducreyi*

■ Appearance

- Very painful erosions and ulcers on the penis or genital area, usually with a gray base

■ Diagnosis
- Scraping base of an ulcer and Gram staining the scrapings: microscopic examination will show gram-negative coccobacilli singly or in "schools of fish."
- Culture of the organism possible, but difficult, as the organism on a swab dies at room temperature within 2 to 4 hours.
- Swabs should be transported quickly to the laboratory or refrigerated.

■ Treatment
- Erythromycin 500 mg po qid for 2 weeks

VIRAL INFECTIONS OF SKIN

Warts (Figure 5-8)

■ Definition
- Wide variety of slow-growing epithelial lesions caused by papillomaviruses
- Include common warts (hands, feet, other cutaneous surfaces), flat warts (face or legs), anogenital warts, cervical warts, laryngeal warts, and perianal warts (condylomata acuminata) that can form large cauliflower-like (exophytic) masses

■ Etiology
- Infection with HPV.
- Different kinds of warts are caused by different strains of HPV. Warts on hands, feet, and face (flat warts) are caused by HPV types 1 to 4, 10, 28, 29, 37, 41, 48, 60, 63, and 65. Warts in the anogenital, cervical, and pharangeal areas are caused by types 6, 11, 30, 34, 40, 42 to 44, 55, and 57 to 59.
- Incidence of warts in immunocompromised patients is greatly increased.

■ Appearance
- Rough, scaly papules occurring singly or in clusters on any skin surface

■ Diagnosis
- Paring of warts will reveal thrombosed capillaries that appear like tiny black dots

■ Treatment
- Liquid nitrogen treatment, topical salicylic acid, topical cantharidin (a blistering agent), or other topical wart preparations.

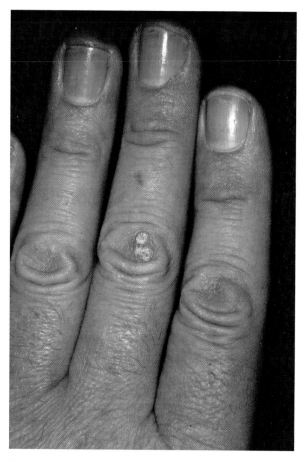

Figure 5-8 • Warts. *(Image courtesy of Dr. Howard Baden, Massachusetts General Hospital/Harvard Medical School, Boston, MA.)*

- Anogenital warts can be treated by painting with podophyllin, which is washed off 6 hours after application. Continued treatment every 2 to 3 weeks is necessary until the wart is completely resolved.
- Immunotherapy using topical immune modulators (e.g., Imiquimod) is useful for treatment of genital warts.
- *Note:* **Some papillomaviruses may affect progression to carcinoma in lesions.**
  - Verrucous carcinoma: low-grade squamous cell carcinoma

- Epithelioma cuniculatum: verrucous carcinoma on plantar surface of the foot
- Bowenoid papulosis: small papules on the external male and female genitalia infected with HPV type 16; histologically shows cellular atypia
- Warts in the anogenital, cervical, and pharangeal areas are sometimes caused by "high-risk" types (16, 18, 31, 33, 35, 39, 45, 51, 52, 56) that may be a factor in carcinogenic progression of some lesions.

Herpes Simplex (Figure 5-9)

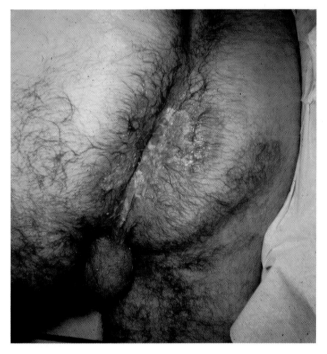

Figure 5-9 • Herpes simplex. *(Image courtesy of Dr. Howard Baden, Massachusetts General Hospital/Harvard Medical School, Boston, MA.)*

■ **Definition**
- Herpes simplex virus infection causing "fever blisters," genital lesions, and other skin lesions, often around the mouth or on the buttocks.

■ **Etiology**
- Herpesvirus I (mouth, skin) or II (genital lesions, skin)

■ **Appearance**
- Clusters of vesicles on erythematous base.
- Vesicle superficial with fragile roof, resulting in erosion.
- Lesions painful with prodrome of stinging and burning.
- Lesions tend to recur in the same areas previously infected.
- Lesions usually resolve in 2 to 3 weeks.
- Virus remains dormant, usually within the trigeminal nerve root ganglion.
- Stress, menstrual periods, illness, and sun exposure can reactivate virus.

■ **Diagnosis**
- Tzanck test: scraping skin from the base of a vesicle, staining with Wright-Giemsa stain, examining for multinucleated "ghost cells" (nuclei of keratinocytes have dissolved)

■ **Treatment**
- Oral acyclovir, valcyclovir, and famcyclovir can shorten course of active infection.
- For those with frequent recurrences, daily suppressive therapy with these medications can lengthen time between attacks.
- *Note:* **Other human herpesvirus that cause infection include varicella zoster virus (shingles), Epstein-Barr virus (Burkitt's lymphoma, infectious mononucleosis), cytomegalovirus (cytomegalovirus inclusion disease), human herpesvirus 6 (exanthem subitum), human herpesvirus 7 (preferentially affects CD4$^+$ lymphocytes), and human herpesvirus 8 (Kaposi's sarcoma).**

Varicella Zoster (Figure 5-10)

■ **Definition**
- Viral infection causing chickenpox and shingles

■ **Etiology**
- Varicella zoster virus, a member of the human herpesvirus family.
- Primary viral infection causes chickenpox.
- After chickenpox, the virus resides (latent) in the sensory nerve ganglia.
- Later in life the virus can be reactivated by a number of factors to result in shingles.

■ **Appearance**
- Chickenpox: prodrome of fever, chills, aching joint, and malaise

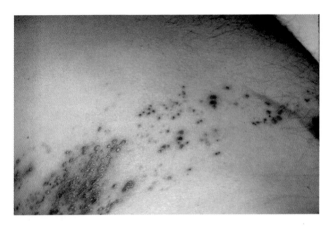

Figure 5-10 • Varicella zoster. *(Image courtesy of Dr. Howard Baden, Massachusetts General Hospital/Harvard Medical School, Boston, MA.)*

- Followed by eruption of widespread erythematous macules and papules that progress to vesicles, then pustules that crust and shed
- Vesicular lesion of chickenpox described as "dewdrop on a rose petal" (Figure 5-11)
- Shingles: painful bullae (large blisters) on an erythematous base in a dermatomal distribution

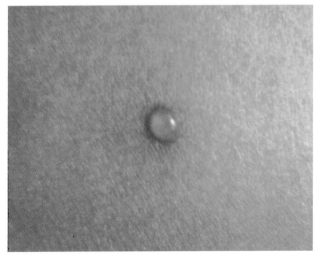

Figure 5-11 • Chickenpox. *(Image courtesy of Dr. Howard Baden, Massachusetts General Hospital/Harvard Medical School, Boston, MA.)*

■ **Diagnosis**

• Tzanck preparation: Scrape skin from base of vesicle, stain with Wright-Giemsa stain, examine for giant cells (intracytoplasmic edema in keratinocytes).

■ **Treatment**

• Oral acyclovir, valcyclovir, or famcyclovir.

• *Note:* Postherpetic neuralgia is a common, but painful, after effect of shingles. The risk for postherpetic neuralgia may be reduced by early treatment with oral antiviral medications.

Molluscum Contagiosum (Figure 5-12)

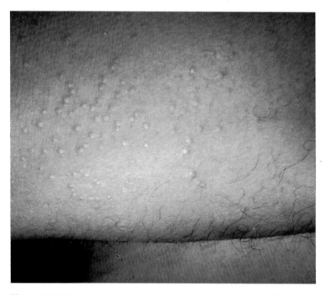

Figure 5-12 • Molluscum contagiosum. *(Image courtesy of Dr. Howard Baden, Massachusetts General Hospital/Harvard Medical School, Boston, MA.)*

■ **Definition**

• Viral disorder transmitted by contact

■ **Etiology**

• Caused by a poxvirus

■ **Appearance**

• Lesions are pink or flesh-colored papules with central umbilication (indentation).

- Often found on young children on arms, legs, and abdomen after contact with other children.
- Sometimes found on adults, often in the lower abdominal area, after contact with a sexual partner.

■ **Diagnosis**
- Usually diagnosed by clinical appearance; biopsy if uncertain as to diagnosis

■ **Treatment**
- Liquid nitrogen, curettage, or application of topical tretinoin (Retin A).
- *Note:* Lesions will eventually resolve on their own. In children with numerous lesions, one option is to not treat, recognizing that additional lesions may occur before resolution occurs.

Insect and Arachnoid Bites

■ **Definition**
- Bites by insects or arachnoids

■ **Etiology**
- Insects (six legs): mosquitos, bees, fleas, fire ants, lice
- Arachnoids (eight legs): mites, spiders

■ **Appearance**
- Typically erythematous papule with a central punctum.
- Lesion can occur singly, in groups, or in linear configurations.
- Occasionally vesicles or hemorrhagic bullae are present.
- Lesion can be extensive, as in the bite of a brown recluse spider: urticaria, bullae, severe necrosis of bite site and surrounding area.
- Can cause a variety of symptoms including itching, stinging and burning, edema, and/or erythema.
- Systemic effects including anaphylaxis can sometimes occur.
- Bites can sometimes result in systemic disease.
- Tick bites can be vectors for disease; bites by certain tick species can result in Lyme disease, erlichiosis, or Rocky Mountain spotted fever with systemic symptoms. Tick bites in some cases can also result in tick paralysis, causing ascending paralysis and potential death, unless the tick is removed. Babesiosis, caused by the intracellular red blood cell parasite *Babesia microti*, can also result from tick bites.
- Scorpion bites and black widow spider bites can result in both local and potentially fatal systemic effects. Bites by some species of caterpillars can also result in severe reactions.

■ **Diagnosis**
- Diagnosis by history; if lice, examine hair for nits (lice eggs).

■ **Treatment**

- Bites that itch can be treated with topical corticosteroid applied twice a day.
- Persistent itching with edema and erythema can be treated with oral antihistamines.
- Severe reactions with edema and difficulty breathing are medical emergencies that require subcutaneous epinephrine (1:1000 solution) injection, corticosteroid injection, and other life support measures.
- Epinephrine emergency kits are available for persons with bee allergy.

Rocky Mountain Spotted Fever (Figure 5-13)

■ **Definition**

- Severe rickettsial disease transmitted by tick bite

■ **Etiology**

- *Rickettsia rickettsii*; usually transmitted by American dog tick (*Dermacentor variabilis*) in eastern United States or Rocky Mountain wood tick (*Dermacentor andersoni*) in western United States

■ **Appearance**

- Fever and chills occur first, followed about 4 days later with an erythematous, maculopapular rash that begins around the wrists, hands, and ankles and spreads centrally to the trunk and upper extremities.
- This central type of spread is in contrast to most infectious rashes that usually begin on the neck and trunk and spread peripherally.
- Petechiae and ecchymoses appear, and diffuse vasculitis develops.
- Areas of gangrene occasionally occur.

■ **Diagnosis**

- Indirect immunofluorescence assay. **Note:** Rocky Mountain spotted fever is a dangerous infection that must be recognized and treated with oral antibiotics. Treatment decisions should be made on clinical and epidemiologic clues and should not be delayed while waiting for confirmation of laboratory results.

■ **Treatment**

- Tetracycline, tetracycline analogs, or chloramphenicol

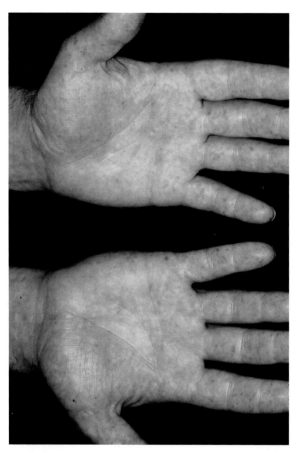

Figure 5-13 • Rocky Mountain spotted fever. *(Image courtesy of Dr. Howard Baden, Massachusetts General Hospital/Harvard Medical School, Boston, MA.)*

PARASITIC INFESTATIONS

Lice

■ **Definition**
- Blood-sucking insects that infest hair-bearing areas (head lice, pubic lice) or live in seams of clothes (body lice)

■ **Etiology**
- *Pediculus humanus capitis:* head louse.

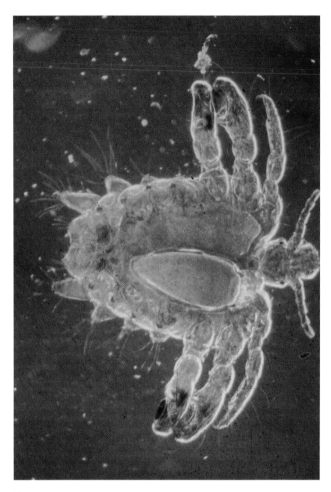

Figure 5-14 • Lice (pubic louse). *(Image courtesy of Dr. Howard Baden, Massachusetts General Hospital/Harvard Medical School, Boston, MA.)*

- *Pthirus pubis:* pubic louse (Figure 5-14).
- *Pediculus humanus corporis:* body louse.
- **Note:** Rarely, lice can transmit epidemic typhus (***Rickettsia prowazekii***), trench fever (***Rickettsia quintana***), and relapsing fever (***Borrelia recurrentis***).

■ Appearance

- Erythematous puncta, sometimes with surrounding erythema.
- Bites can be pruritic (itchy) and/or painful.
- There may be only a few lice or hundreds.

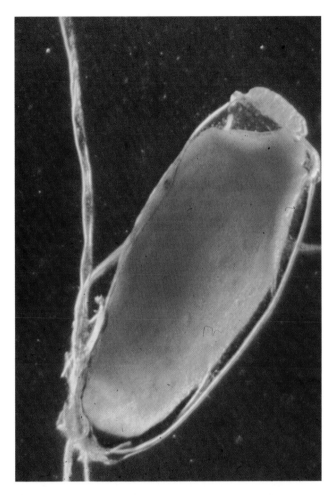

Figure 5-15 • Lice (nit). *(Image courtesy of Dr. Howard Baden, Massachusetts General Hospital/Harvard Medical School, Boston, MA.)*

■ Diagnosis

- Clinical examination of scalp and clothes for lice
- Examination of scalp for nits (white dots on hair shaft)
- Microscopic examination of nits (eggs glued to hair shafts) (Figure 5-15) to confirm diagnosis

■ Treatment

- Lice can be difficult to eradicate.
- For hair-bearing areas infested with lice, use permethrin (Nix) shampoo or pyrethrin (Rid) shampoo.

- Follow shampoo with vinegar rinse and fine-toothed combing to remove nits.
- For treatment of skin infested with body lice, use lindane (Kwell) or permethrins (Elimite).
- Clothes of patients with body lice should be cleaned and ironed.
- Sulfur (4%–10%) in petrolatum can also be applied to skin or scalp infested with lice.
- *Note:* Lice infestation can quickly spread through a classroom of children, and children with nits should not attend class until treatment has been started. The CDC recommends that an infested child be kept from a child-care setting until 24 hours after treatment has started. Many states and local health departments require that the child be free of nits before readmission to school or child care. Children should be checked daily for evidence of new or continued infection for 10 days after treatment. Retreatment in 7 to 10 days may be necessary.

Scabies (Figure 5-16)

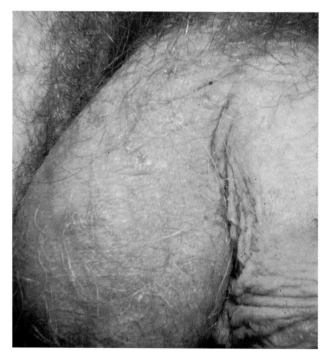

Figure 5-16 • Scabies. *(Image courtesy of Dr. Howard Baden, Massachusetts General Hospital/Harvard Medical School, Boston, MA.)*

■ **Definition**
- Scabies mites are arthropods that live, lay eggs within the skin (stratum corneum), and bite.

■ **Etiology**
- *Sarcoptes scabiei*, variation hominis

■ **Appearance**
- Scaly papules and excoriations (from scratching) as well as tiny linear or wavy "burrows" in warm areas such as between fingers and toes, in the umbilicus, around the waistline, and on the penile shaft.
- Skin infested with scabies is extremely itchy.

■ **Diagnosis**
- Microscopic examination of papule, erosion, or burrow for scabies (six-legged) mite, mite eggs, or mite feces

■ **Treatment**
- Lindane (Kwell) or permethrin (Elimite) applied from the neck down, left on overnight, and washed off the following morning; repeat procedure 1 week later.
- The morning after treatment, launder sheets, bedclothes, and towels.
- Entire family should be treated in confirmed cases.
- Sulfur (4%–10%) in petrolatum can also be used to treat skin infested with scabies.
- *Note:* **Infestation with hundreds of mites is called Norwegian scabies and can occur in nursing home patients or otherwise debilitated patients. Oral ivermectin (single dose of 200 µg/kg body weight) alone or combined with topical treatment has been successful in treating patients with Norwegian scabies.**

6 Skin Manifestations of Systemic Disorders

Skin often gives clues as to what is going on systemically. For example, liver disorders (hepatitis) can cause color changes in skin and itching. Disorders that affect vasculature (e.g., cryoglobulinemia, diabetes, polyarteritis) can cause skin ulcers. Metastasis of internal carcinomas often manifest first on the skin as tumorous growths. Viral disorders, disseminated bacterial or fungal infection, and drug reactions can cause rashes.

SKIN MANIFESTATIONS OF SYSTEMIC VIRAL INFECTIONS

- Some viral infections can result in rash as well as usual symptoms of a cold.
- The rash may be maculopapular, may involve trunk and extremities, and often involves palms and soles.
- The rash may precede, accompany, or follow other symptoms.
- When palms or soles are involved, think of viral infection.
- *Note:* Syphilis (spirochetal), erythema multiforme (hypersensitivity reaction), and Rocky Mountain spotted fever (rickettsial) can also involve palms and soles.

Erythema Infectiosum ("Fifth Disease")

■ Definition
- Systemic viral infection with rash

■ Etiology
- Parvovirus B19, thought to be transmitted by respiratory route.
- Most infectious time is prior to development of rash.

■ Appearance
- Erythematous or "slapped cheeks."
- Systemic symptoms of coryza, headache, fever, and malaise occur first, followed by erythematous, macular rash on the trunk and extensor surfaces of extremities.

■ **Diagnosis**

- Clinical picture is usually sufficient; if necessary, one can confirm findings with IgM assays or *in situ* hybridization.

■ **Treatment**

- Symptomatic treatment.
- *Note:* **Fetal hydrops with extensive hemolysis can occur in a fetus infected with this virus.**

HIV Disease

■ **Definition**

- Systemic viral infection that predisposes affected individuals to a wide variety of skin as well as systemic disorders.

■ **Etiology**

- HIV virus

■ **Appearance**

- Viral and fungal diseases are especially common in AIDS patients and include huge condyloma accuminata (very large anal wart clusters caused by human papillomavirus), numerous molluscum contagiosum, and deep fungal infections such as blastomycosis, coccidioidomycosis, and histoplasmosis.
- Herpes simplex virus and varicella zoster virus infections are also common (may be systemic symptoms as well as cutaneous).
- A sudden onset of seborrheic dermatitis or psoriasis should raise suspicion of HIV disease.
- Pruritic folliculitis or pruritus in general is common in HIV disease.
- See index for reference to descriptions of these disorders in this book.

■ **Diagnosis**

- HIV serology
- Biopsy of skin lesions not clinically diagnostic

■ **Treatment**

- UV treatment can be helpful for pruritus.
- Condyloma can be treated with liquid nitrogen or podophillin.
- Molluscum can be treated with liquid nitrogen.
- Deep fungal infections should be treated with systemic antifungals such as amphotericin.
- Herpes simplex virus and varicella zoster virus infections are treated with antiviral medications such as acyclovir (herpes

simplex: acyclovir 400 mg tid; varicella zoster virus: acyclovir 800 mg five times per day). Intravenous acyclovir (5–10 mg/kg tid) may be necessary for resistant cases.

SKIN MANIFESTATIONS OF SYSTEMIC BACTERIAL INFECTIONS

Scarlet Fever

■ **Definition**

• Disease with diffuse erythematous rash, usually occurring in children, characterized by sore throat and fever, followed by enlarged, red tonsils, lymphadenopathy, and white-coated tongue with red protruding papillae ("white-strawberry" tongue)

■ **Etiology**

• Circulating toxin produced by group A streptococcus

■ **Appearance**

• Diffuse maculopapular rash on the trunk and extremities, flushed cheeks, and circumoral pallor.
• Desquamation begins as soon as the rash begins to fade.
• May be petechiae in a linear configuration in the antecubital fossae and axillary folds, often termed Pastia's lines.

■ **Diagnosis**

• Culture for streptococcus infection

■ **Treatment**

• Penicillin

Syphilis (Figure 6-1)

■ **Definition**

• Sexually transmitted disease causing rash and systemic symptoms

■ **Etiology**

• Caused by spirochete (*Treponema pallidum*)
• Transmitted by sexual contact with an infected partner, prenatally from an infected mother, by direct inoculation (laboratory workers), or by transfusion (rare)

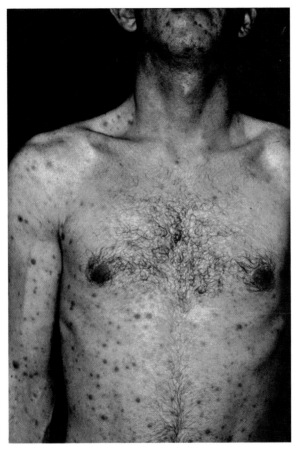

Figure 6-1 • Syphilis. *(Image courtesy of Dr. Howard Baden, Massachusetts General Hospital/Harvard Medical School, Boston, MA.)*

■ Appearance
- Often called, "the great imitator" because rash produced can take many forms.
- Classically painless chancre (primary lesion) appears as ulcerated nodule at site of sexual innoculation, followed a couple of months later by secondary stage, a nonpruritic rash that covers the trunk and extremities.
- Rash typically consists of small erythematous macules that progress into erythematous papules or oval plaques with scale.
- Dark, copper-colored macules often found on palms and soles.

- Mucous patches in mouth.
- May be alopecia with "moth-eaten" appearance.
- In third stage of syphilis, systemic problems can occur such as hepatitis, gastritis, arthritis, and renal disease.
- Neurosyphilis as well as cardiovascular syphilis can rarely occur.
- Cardiovascular syphilis often includes aortic valvular disease.
- Prior to development of antibiotics, syphilis was major cause of death due to aortic rupture.
- Late manifestations of syphilis include gummas, which appear as large tumorous swellings, often ulcerated, and may be seen in different organs.

■ **Diagnosis**
- Dark-field microscopic examination for spirochetes

■ **Treatment**
- Two intramuscular injections (1 week apart) of 2.4 million units benzathine penicillin G.
- Contacts must be determined and treated.
- If not treated, syphilis can result in cardiac, osteopathic, and neurologic complications.
- Offspring of an infected, untreated woman have a high risk for congenital syphilis.
- *Note:* **Cases of syphilis must be reported to the local health department, where treatment and follow-up of contacts is conducted.**

SKIN MANIFESTATION OF RICKETTSIAL INFECTIONS

See Chapter 5 for discussion of Rocky Mountain spotted fever.

SKIN MANIFESTATION OF DEEP FUNGAL INFECTIONS

- Examples of deep fungal infections include sporotrichosis, blastomycosis, chromoblastomycosis, coccidioidomycosis, aspergillosis, mycetoma, histoplasmosis, paracoccidioidomycosis, alternarianosis, rhinosporidiosis, geotrichosis, lobomycosis, actinomycosis, nocardiosis, allescheria, mucormycosis, and cryptococcosis.
- Inflammatory nodules or plaques with ulceration, crust, and exudate should arouse suspicion of a deep fungal infection.
- Since these diseases are fairly rare in the general population, they are not discussed here.
- Deep fungal infections are more likely to be seen in the AIDS population.

METABOLIC DISORDERS WITH SKIN MANIFESTATIONS

Porphyria

■ **Definition**
- Inherited metabolic disorder that results from defects in enzyme activity in the heme synthesis pathway

■ **Etiology**
- Porphyrins are intermediates in heme synthesis; when the heme synthesis pathway is blocked, porphyria results.
- Major source of excess porphyrins in erythropoietic protoporphyria and congenital erythropoietic porphyria is skin.
- Major source of excess porphyrins in acute intermittent porphyria, aminolevulinic acid (ALA) dehydratase porphyria, porphyria cutanea tarda, variegate porphyria, and hereditary coproporphyria is liver.

■ **Appearance**
- There are different types of porphyria with different symptoms, depending on where the pathway is blocked.
- Skin changes occur in porphyria cutanea tarda (skin fragility), erythropoietic protoporphyria, congenital erythropoietic porphyria, variegate porphyria, and sometimes in hereditary coproporphyria.
- Congenital erythropoietic porphyria: pink urine and marked photosensitivity, blistering and crusted erosions on sun exposed areas, photosensitivity delayed.
- Erythropoietic protoporphyria: immediate phototoxicity with stinging, burning, erythema of skin; sun-exposed skin becomes thickened and leathery.
- Porphyria cutanea tarda: facial hypertrichosis and easy fragility of skin, delayed-type hypersensitivity with bullae, erosions, scarring; also associated with chronic renal failure, alcoholism, and hepatitis.
- Hereditary coproporphyria: photosensitivity (30% of cases) similar to that found in porphyria cutanea tarda.
- Variegate porphyria: may have cutaneous manifestations of photosensitivity.
- Certain medications should not be taken by persons with porphyria since they will exacerbate the condition.

■ **Diagnosis**
- Urine and stool to laboratory to check for porphyrins

■ **Treatment**
- Sunscreen use is important for patients with porphyria.
- Phlebotomy often helpful: Remove approximately 500 mL of whole blood each week, or twice a week, monitoring hemoglobin carefully to maintain above 11 or 12 g/dL.

SYSTEMIC DISORDERS WITH SKIN MANIFESTATIONS AND UNKNOWN ETIOLOGY

Kawasaki's Disease

■ **Definition**
- Acute, vascular disease of unknown etiology that occurs during childhood

■ **Etiology**
- Unknown

■ **Appearance**
- "Cherry red lips," "strawberry tongue" (hyperemia, hypertrophic papillae).
- Prolonged high fever, followed by a morbilliform eruption on the trunk and extremities.
- Erythematous, desquamating rash on the perineum.
- Conjunctival infection usually present.
- Often edema and erythema of the hands and feet.
- Myocarditis, pericardial effusion, coronary artery aneurysms can occur.

■ **Diagnosis**
- Diagnosis by clinical presentation

■ **Treatment**
- Single, high dose of intravenous gammaglobulin (2 g/kg) and high-dose aspirin (80–100 mg/kg per day) useful

Pyoderma Gangrenosum (Figure 6-2)

■ **Definition**
- Painful nodule or pustule, solitary or multiple, forming a progressively enlarging ulcer

■ **Etiology**
- May be present without underlying disorder or may be associated with systemic diseases such as Crohn's disease, ulcerative cholitis, polyarthritis, leukemias, and monoclonal gammopathy

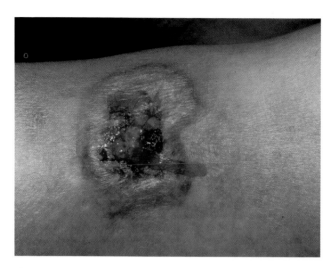

Figure 6-2 • Pyoderma gangrenosum. *(Image courtesy of Dr. Howard Baden, Massachusetts General Hospital/Harvard Medical School, Boston, MA.)*

■ **Appearance**
• Irregular ulcer with raised, overhanging, inflammatory border and boggy, necrotic base

■ **Diagnosis**
• Clinical appearance.
• "Pathergy" often present; new lesions develop or old lesions expand with trivial trauma.
• Histopathologic features not diagnostic.

■ **Treatment**
• Treatment of any underlying disorder
• Systemic corticosteroids or other immunosuppressive therapy

HYPERSENSITIVITY REACTIONS

Atopic Dermatitis (Eczema) (Figure 6-3)

See also section on Eczema in Chapter 3.

■ **Definition**
• Chronic disorder that usually begins in childhood

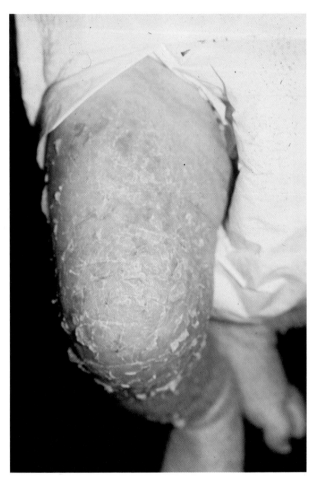

Figure 6-3 · Atopic dermatitis and eczema. *(Image courtesy of Dr. Howard Baden, Massachusetts General Hospital/Harvard Medical School, Boston, MA.)*

■ **Etiology**
- Often associated with a family history of atopic dermatitis and a personal history of other atopic diseases such as food allergies and asthma.

■ **Appearance**
- Erythematous papules, plaques, and excoriations.
- Extremely pruritic.

- Superimposed infection with *Staphylococcus* or *Streptococcus* often occurs.
- In babies, lesions of atopic dermatitis are often found on lateral aspects of arms and on cheeks.
- As the child becomes old enough to scratch, lesions are found in the antecubital fossae, on the abdomen, and in the posterior fossae.

■ **Diagnosis**
- Diagnosis by clinical presentation

■ **Treatment**
- Use of mild, unscented soaps and moisturizers.
- Avoidance of perfumed products.
- Application of mild topical corticosteroids.
- Topical tacrolimus (FK506, Protopic) sometimes helpful.
- Oral antibiotics often necessary when superinfection of eroded skin occurs.
- Affected child will sometimes outgrow this condition at puberty.
- Condition will sometimes linger into adulthood.
- ***Note: Eczema* is a general term sometimes used to refer to atopic dermatitis, but also to other conditions caused by irritation of skin by scratching or by a variety of substances, such as perfumed lotions or soaps, dish detergent, exposure to nickel, or exposure to other irritants or allergans. Eczema is treated with topical corticosteroids or with topical tacrolimus. It is important to emphasize to patients the importance of use of mild, unscented soaps and unscented moisturizers, as well as avoidance of irritating substances in daily skin care.**

Urticaria (Figure 6-4)

■ **Definition**
- Skin (and sometimes systemic) manifestation of an allergic reaction

■ **Etiology**
- Allergic reaction.
- Many things can precipitate urticaria in sensitized persons: e.g., foods, medicines, viral disorders (especially hepatitis B), helminth infections, autoimmune disorders such as lupus, among others.

■ **Appearance**
- Red wheals that "come and go" (lesions appear in one place, fade, appear in another place) on parts of body and cause severe itching.

Figure 6-4 · Urticaria. *(Image courtesy of Dr. Howard Baden, Massachusetts General Hospital/Harvard Medical School, Boston, MA.)*

- Lips and face may be swollen.
- In severe cases, breathing can become compromised, resulting in an emergency.

■ **Diagnosis**
- Good history taking most important.
- May be helpful in determining cause to screen for hepatitis, check stool for ova and parasites, obtain blood work, and check for antinuclear antibodies (ANA)
- Especially important to ask about recent antibiotic use, especially penicillin or sulfa medications.

- Some people may develop urticaria to nuts, chocolate, fried foods, or beer.

■ **Treatment**

- Elimination of offending factor, if determined.
- Oral antihistamines.
- Avoid all irritating substances.
- Use only mild, unscented soap for bathing.
- Apply moisturizer after bathing.
- In cases where sensitivity to food of some kind is suspected, but the actual food to which the patient is reacting cannot be determined, bland diet such as rice and tea may be helpful in resolving the urticaria. Food groups can then be added back one at a time.
- In severe cases of urticaria, injection of corticosteroids will give temporary relief but should not be relied on for standard therapy since urticaria can be a chronic condition and since there could be underlying problems that corticosteroids could exacerbate.
- *Important:* Patients with urticaria should be warned to seek immediate medical emergency treatment if difficulty with breathing occurs.

Fixed Drug Eruption (Figure 6-5)

■ **Definition**

- Hypersensitivity reaction to one of many medications (e.g., sulfonamides, metronidazole, tetracycline, minocycline, fiorinal, naproxen, salicylates, oral contraceptives, phenacetin, barbitrates, phenolphthalein, among others)

■ **Etiology**

- Hypersensitivity skin reaction

■ **Appearance**

- Single or several sharply demarcated, erythematous patches.
- With rechallenge of drug, the lesion occurs in the same location.

■ **Diagnosis**

- Clinical picture
- Biopsy

■ **Treatment**

- Elimination of precipitant cause

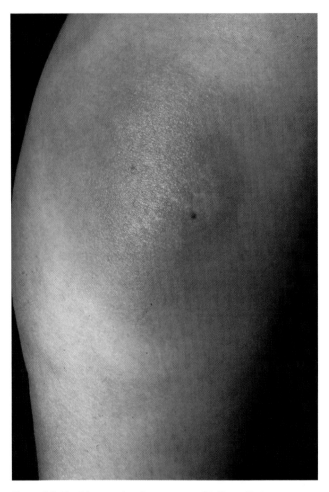

Figure 6-5 · Fixed drug reaction. *(Image courtesy of Dr. Howard Baden, Massachusetts General Hospital/Harvard Medical School, Boston, MA.)*

ERYTHEMA MULTIFORME, STEVENS-JOHNSON SYNDROME, AND TOXIC EPIDERMAL NECROLYSIS

Erythema Multiforme Minor (Figure 6-6)

■ Definition

• Erythema multiforme minor: hypersensitivity skin reaction to one of many precipitating factors, including viral disorders (e.g., herpes simplex) and medications (e.g., sulfa drugs)

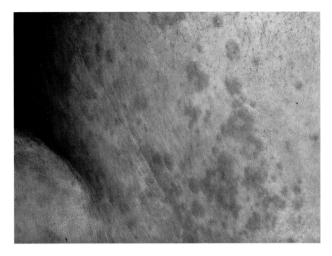

Figure 6-6 · Erythema multiforme. *(Image courtesy of Dr. Howard Baden, Massachusetts General Hospital/Harvard Medical School, Boston, MA.)*

■ **Etiology**
- Hypersensitivity skin reaction

■ **Appearance**
- Erythema multiforme minor: "Target" lesions (macules, edematous papules consisting of concentric rings) can be found on palms, soles, trunk, and extremities.
- Concentric rings: usually a central area of dusky erythema surrounded by a lighter, edematous ring and an outside ring of erythema.
- Histologically there is spongiosis, clusters of necrotic keratinocytes, and perivascular infiltrate of lymphocytes.

■ **Diagnosis**
- Biopsy if not clinically diagnostic

■ **Treatment**
- Eliminate the precipitant cause, if detected.
- Treat symptomatically.
- Systemic antihistamines are usually helpful.
- Follow patients carefully to monitor for tendency toward progression to the more severe Stevens-Johnson syndrome (erythema multiforme major).

Erythema Multiforme Major
(Stevens-Johnson Syndrome)

■ **Definition**
- A severe mucocutaneous form of erythema multiforme

■ **Etiology**
- Severe hypersensitivity reaction

■ **Appearance**
- Erosions and bullae on skin and mucous membranes, especially in and around mouth
- Painful, widespread purpuric macules; some detachment of the epidermis
- Severe mucous membrane involvement with heavy crusting of lips

■ **Diagnosis**
- Careful history of medications; test for herpes, *Mycoplasma*, other infections.

■ **Treatment**
- Elimination of the precipitant cause
- Supportive therapy

Toxic Epidermal Necrolysis (TEN) (Figure 6-7)

■ **Definition**
- Hypersensitivity reaction at the severe end of the erythema multiforme/Stevens-Johnson spectrum

■ **Etiology**
- Severe hypersensitivity reaction
- Precipitating factors similar to those of Stevens-Johnson syndrome and erythema multiforme
- Sulfa drugs and phenytoin (dilantin) frequently implicated in TEN

■ **Appearance**
- Body reacts severely, shedding entire epidermis of skin in sheets, causing fluid loss and severe risk of superimposed bacterial infection.
- Nikolsky's sign is present (blisters spread with pressure, indicating easy separation of the epidermis from underlying dermis).

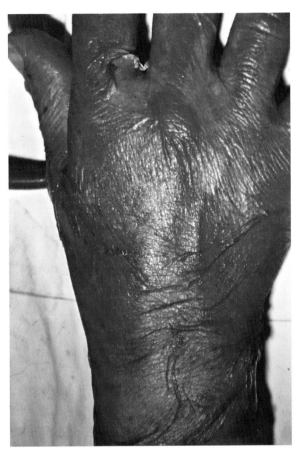

Figure 6-7 • Toxic epidermal necrolysis. *(Image courtesy of Dr. Howard Baden, Massachusetts General Hospital/Harvard Medical School, Boston, MA.)*

■ **Diagnosis**
• Monitor laboratory results and fluids. If infection suspected, culture blood and other body fluids.

■ **Treatment**
• Patient should be placed in the burn unit of the hospital for treatment.
• Severe condition with high mortality rate.

Erythema Nodosum

See Chapter 3 for description of erythema nodosum.

Graft-Versus-Host Disease

■ **Definition**
- Transplanted, competent immune cells react against cells in an immunocompromised host following transplantation (including bone marrow transplantation).

■ **Etiology**
- Immune reaction of host cells against donor cells

■ **Appearance**
- Affects skin, gastrointestinal tract, and liver.
- Erythematous macules develop on hands, feet, and pinnae of ears, spreading to the trunk and extremities.
- Rarely the macules develop into plaques or bullae.
- Histologically the rash is characterized by vacuolar changes in the basal layer of the epidermis and dyskeratotic keratinocytes in the epidermis.

■ **Diagnosis**
- Monitor for infection.
- Supportive treatment.

■ **Treatment**
- Treatment with corticosteroids or other immunosuppressants.
- Prophylactic treatment with methotrexate or cyclosporine prior to bone marrow infusion after bone marrow transplantation will reduce incidence of graft-versus-host disease.

Canker Sores (Figure 6-8)

■ **Definition**
- Aphthous ulcers (mouth ulcers)

■ **Etiology**
- Often associated with stress, illness, menses, or other factors
- Sometimes associated with coxsackie virus (herpangina; hand, foot, and mouth disease), Stevens-Johnson syndrome (discussed previously), Behçet's disease (ulcers of oral and genital mucosa; eye disease, vasculitis, arthritis), Reiter's syndrome (urethritis, arthritis, conjunctivitis), and other diseases

■ **Appearance**
- Painful ulcers in mouth
- White erosions on erythematous base

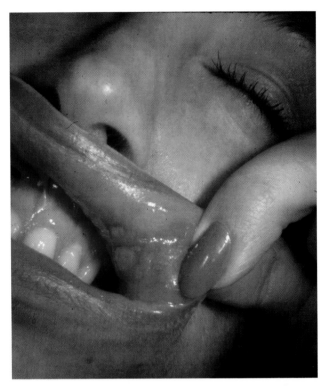

Figure 6-8 · Aphthous ulcers (canker sores). *(Image courtesy of Dr. Howard Baden, Massachusetts General Hospital/Harvard Medical School, Boston, MA.)*

■ **Diagnosis**
• Clinical appearance

■ **Treatment**
• Symptomatic treatment with swish and spit solutions (equal parts tetracycline, lidocaine, and diphenhydramine HCl [Benadryl]) or with topically applied corticosteroids

HYPERSENSITIVITY DISORDERS OF PREGNANCY

Pruritic Urticarial Papules of Pregnancy (Figure 6-9)

■ **Definition**
• Hypersensitivity reaction during pregnancy

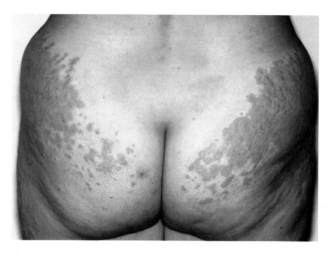

Figure 6-9 · Pruritic urticarial papules of pregnancy. *(Image courtesy of Dr. Howard Baden, Massachusetts General Hospital/Harvard Medical School, Boston, MA.)*

■ **Etiology**
• Hypersensitivity reaction

■ **Appearance**
• Pruritic eruption of erythematous and edematous papules, typically developing on the trunk and extremities during the third trimester of pregnancy
• Histologically: edema in the papillary dermis and perivascular infiltrate of lymphocytes, monocytes, and eosinophils

■ **Diagnosis**
• Biopsy if in doubt of diagnosis

■ **Treatment**
• Oral antihistamines, emollients, and topical corticosteroids can be helpful if rash extensive and uncomfortable.
• Tapering dose of corticosteroids may be necessary for severe cases.
• Rash will usually resolve after delivery of the baby.
• Co-manage with patient's obstetrician to monitor laboratory results, blood pressure, and status of infant, especially if giving oral corticosteroids. ***Warning:* Oral corticosteroids can cause high blood pressure and premature rupture of the uterine membrane.**

Herpes Gestationis (Figure 6-10)

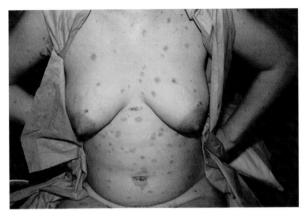

Figure 6-10 • Herpes gestationis. *(Image courtesy of Dr. Howard Baden, Massachusetts General Hospital/Harvard Medical School, Boston, MA.)*

■ **Definition**
- Autoimmune disorder that occurs during pregnancy or immediately following pregnancy

■ **Etiology**
- Autoimmune disorder
- *Not* caused by herpesvirus

■ **Appearance**
- Bullae and vesicles on an erythematous base
- Annular or serpentiginous lesions composed of bullae or vesicles that extend over the abdomen, to other parts of the trunk, and to extremities
- Rash extremely pruritic

■ **Diagnosis**
- Biopsy for histopathology and immunofluorescence if in doubt of diagnosis

■ **Treatment**
- Oral antihistamines and oral corticosteroids if necessary for comfort.
- Presence of this disorder does not appear to pose significant risk to the fetus.
- Co-manage with patient's obstetrician to monitor laboratory results, blood pressure, and status of infant, especially if giving

oral corticosteroids. *Warning:* Oral corticosteroids can cause high blood pressure and premature rupture of the uterine membrane.

AUTOIMMUNE REACTIONS

- Collagen-vascular diseases and other autoimmune reactions can result in rash or other skin changes.
- Examples of such disorders include dermatomyositis, lupus, and scleroderma.

Dermatomyositis

■ **Definition**

- Autoimmune disorder characterized by rash and progressive, proximal muscle weakness.

■ **Etiology**

- Unknown

■ **Appearance**

- Erythematous papules (Gottron's papules) over digits of the fingers and metatarsophalangeal joints.
- Periorbital erythema.
- Maculopapular rash in a "shawl-like" distribution on upper back and upper arms.
- Calcium deposits are often noted in children.
- Underlying malignancy sometimes is associated with dermatomyositis in adults.

■ **Diagnosis**

- Biopsy for histology: vacuolar degeneration of basal cells, atrophy of epidermis, degeneration of basement membrane, necrosis in muscle fibers
- Laboratory studies: serum muscle enzymes (creatinine phosphokinase) often elevated, ANA, anti-Jo-1
- Electromyogram of symptomatic (weak, sore) muscles usually abnormal

■ **Treatment**

- Oral corticosteroids or other immunosuppressive treatment

Lupus (Figure 6-11)

■ **Definition**

- Autoimmune disorder characterized by development of antibodies to skin and other organs

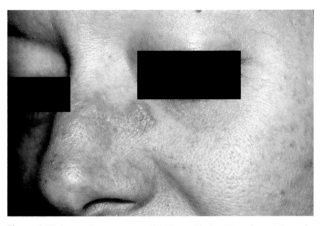

Figure 6-11 • Lupus. *(Image courtesy of Dr. Howard Baden, Massachusetts General Hospital/Harvard Medical School, Boston, MA.)*

■ **Etiology**
• Unknown

■ **Appearance**
• Erythematous patches and papules between the digits of the fingers and over the malar area of the face.
• Photosensitivity
• Oral ulcers
• Discoid lesions on face and extremities (Figure 6-12). Discoid lesions are erythematous lesions with well-defined borders that heal with atrophy and scarring.

■ **Diagnosis**
• Biopsy for histology: vacuolar changes at the basement membrane, necrotic keratinocytes, lymphocytic infiltration of basement membrane zone, thickening basement membrane.
• Laboratory studies: positive ANA, positive anti-double-stranded ANA.

■ **Treatment**
• Topical corticosteroids or antimalarials (hydroxychloroquine 200–400 mg per day, chloroquine 250 mg per day, or quinacrine 100 mg per day).
• *Note:* It is important for the patient to have a baseline ophthalmologic examination prior to starting antimalarials, as well as periodic eye examinations.
• *Note:* Medications such as hydralazine, procainamide, isoniazid, chloromazine, and methyldopa can sometimes induce lupus.

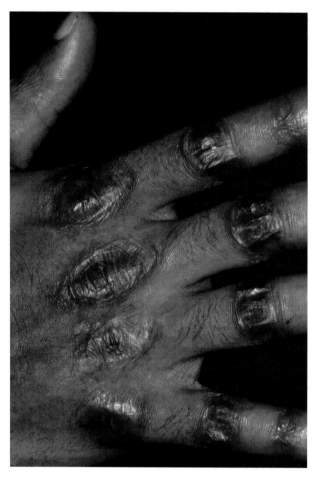

Figure 6-12 · Discoid lupus. *(Image courtesy of Dr. Howard Baden, Massachusetts General Hospital/Harvard Medical School, Boston, MA.)*

Scleroderma

See also section on Scleroderma in Chapter 3.

■ **Definition**
• Autoimmune disorder characterized by tightening of skin

■ **Etiology**
• Unknown

■ **Appearance**

- Thickening and tightening of skin of fingers (sclerodactyly), hands, face, neck, and trunk
- Digital pitting scars
- History of Raynaud's phenomenon (fingers turn blue, then red with cold)

■ **Diagnosis**

- X-ray: bibasilar pulmonary fibrosis
- Biopsy for histology: perivascular infiltration of lymphocytes, plasma cells around vessels, thickened collagen bundles of the dermis
- Laboratory studies: positive ANA

■ **Treatment**

- Calcium channel blocker (to prevent new digit ulceration), colchicine, D-Penicillamine, or oral corticosteroids.
- Interferon-gamma, cyclosporine, or extracorporeal photochemotherapy may be helpful.
- Refer to specialist for treatment.

PARANEOPLASTIC SYNDROMES

- Skin often offers clues to underlying malignancies.
- Some syndromes warn of occult or developing carcinomas.
- See Table 6-1 for examples of paraneoplastic syndromes.
- Workup for carcinoma is warranted if these conditions are present.

GENETIC DISORDERS

- There are many inherited conditions affecting skin and other organs
- Skin often gives clue to underlying genetic conditions.
- No current treatments for these disorders other than symptomatic treatment.

Tuberous Sclerosis

■ **Definition**

- Multisystem, hereditary disorder with fibrous lesions in skin, heart (rhabdomyoma), nervous system (brain "tubers" [sclerosis]), kidney (hamartomas), eye (retinal gliomas [phakomas]), lungs (cysts and fibrosis), and other organs.
- Patients often are mentally retarded and have seizures.

■ TABLE 6-1 Paraneoplastic Conditions

Condition	Clinical Presentation	Association
Sweet's syndrome (reactive process, not an infiltration of leukemia cells); sometimes called "acute febrile neutrophilic dermatosis"	Tender plaques and nodules with erythema, vesicles, and pustules, usually located on extremities or face	Myelocytic leukemia
Subcutaneous fat necrosis	Inflammatory nodules of ulcers on lower extremities and buttocks	Acinar cell adenocarcinoma of pancreas; also associated with pancreatitis or pancreatic pseudocyst
Dermatomyositis	Promixal muscle weakness of upper and lower extremities, heliotrope rash (periorbital edema and erythema), Gottron's papules (erythematous papules over finger digits), often erythematous maculopapular rash in "shawl" distribution on upper chest, upper arms, upper back	Occult or developing bronchogenic carcinoma or cancer of breast, ovary, or cervix
Acanthosis nigricans	Dark brown velvety thickening of skin of axilla, neck, hands, or other areas or of skin	Can be benign condition, often associated with obesity, can be a marker for a number of malignancies, especially gastric adenocarcinoma
Flushing	Facial flushing, abdominal pain, diarrhea (normal flushing can occur with exercise, heat, some foods, and hormonal changes)	Carcinoid syndrome
Erythema gyratum repens	Rapidly migrating eruption with erythematous, annular plaques that give a "wood-grain" appearance.	Carcinoma of esophagus, stomach, bladder, prostate, breast, lung, or cervix
Necrolytic migratory erythema ("glucogonoma syndrome")	Erythematous plaques, erosions, pustules, bullae; also on central face, especially around the mouth	Glucagonoma
Acrokeratosis of Bazex	Erythema and scale on nose, ears, feet, around nails, cheeks, trunk	Cancer of upper respiratory tract

■ **Etiology**

- Genetic disorder transmitted by autosomal-dominant inheritance with variable expression.
- Mutations of genes on a portion of chromosome 9 and 16 may be involved.
- Multiple genes may play a role.

■ **Appearance**

- Pink or red angiofibromas usually located on the cheeks and chin (adenoma sebaceum)
- Hypopigmented macules ("ash-leaf"spots)
- Slightly elevated plaques of subepidermal fibrosis with a rough "orange-peel" surface appearance (shagreen patch)
- Fibromas under or around the fingernails or toenails (Koenen's tumors)
- Brown patches (café au lait spots)
- Soft fibromas

■ **Diagnosis**

- Clinical evaluation: The Diagnostic Criteria Committee of the National Tuberous Sclerosis Association has developed diagnostic criteria helpful in diagnosing this disorder.
- Biopsy to confirm angiofibroma.

■ **Treatment**

- Monitor for medical complications.
- Genetic counseling (50% of children with affected parent are at risk).
- Angiofibromas of the face or periungual fibromas, if troublesome cosmetically, can be treated surgically or with laser.

Neurofibromatosis (Figure 6-13)

■ **Definition**

- Multisystem disorder, inherited or acquired by spontaneous mutation

■ **Etiology**

- Approximately half of patients with neurofibromatosis inherit the disorder: another half develop the disorder spontaneously.
- NF1: caused by mutations in the NF1 gene, located on the long arm of chromosome 17; there is variable expressivity of the gene, and many different mutations have been described.
- NF2: caused by mutations in the NF2 gene, located on chromosome 22.

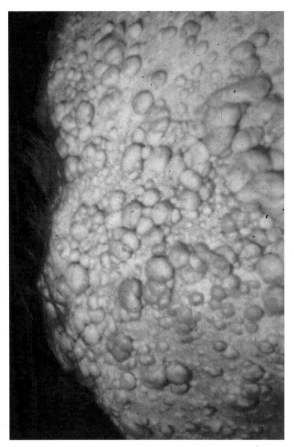

Figure 6-13 · Neurofibromatosis. *(Image courtesy of Dr. Howard Baden, Massachusetts General Hospital/Harvard Medical School, Boston, MA.)*

■ **Appearance**

- There are many different types of neurofibromatosis with varying clinical manifestations and different inheritance patterns.
- Neurofibromas (flesh-colored, soft papules and nodules), café au lait spots, axillary freckling, and hamartomatous lesions of bone and central nervous system.
- NF1: large number of neurofibromas, including plexiform (very large) lesions, optic gliomas, iris hamartomas, dysplasia of the sphenoid bone, thinning of the cortex of long bones.
- More than six café au lait macules (hyperpigmented macules larger than 1.5 cm) confers a presumptive diagnosis of NF1, as

does having a first-degree relative with NF1 or finding any one of a number of other characteristics, including presence of axillary or inguinal freckling, two or more neurofibromas or one plexiform neurofibroma, two or more Lisch's nodules, optic glioma, or thinning of the long bone cortex.

- NF2 has only a few skin abnormalities, which include neurofibromas and schwannomas. Bilateral acoustic neurofibromas can be found, as can meningiomas, gliomas, schwannomas, and juvenile posterior cataracts.

■ **Diagnosis**

- Biopsy of neurofibroma.
- NF1: monitor for optic gliomas.
- NF2: periodic MRI of head to monitor for bilateral acoustic neuromas.

■ **Treatment**

- Management of neurofibromatosis, like other hereditary disorders, consists of monitoring for medical complications.

TABLE 6-2 Other Genetic Disorders with Skin Abnormalities	
Basal cell nevus syndrome	Frequent development of basal cell carcinomas and jaw cysts
Xeroderma pigmentosum	Defects in repair of damage from ultraviolet radiation and development of numerous skin cancers incuding squamous cell carcinoma and melanoma
Porphyria (inherited or acquired)	Deficiency in heme biosynthesis pathway; photosensitivity
Pseudoxanthoma elasticum	Abnormalities of connective tissue, development of "cobblestone appearing" skin and elastic tissue calcification
Ehlers-Danlos syndrome	Hyperelastic skin and poor wound healing
Incontinentia pigmenti	Vesiculobullous eruption at birth, followed by verrucous lesions that transition into whorled slate gray macular pigmentation on the trunk and extremities
Ectodermal dysplasias	Abnormal development of hair, teeth, nails, sweat glands, skin, eyes, and ears
Ichthyoses	Disorders affecting the cornified layer of skin

- Change in size or character of a plexiform neurofibroma suggests possible malignant transformation.
- Genetic counseling: half of the children of a patient with NF1 are at risk for developing NF1.

Other genetic disorders with skin abnormalities are outlined in Table 6-2.

7 Benign and Malignant Growths

BENIGN GROWTHS

Moles (Nevi) (Figure 7-1)

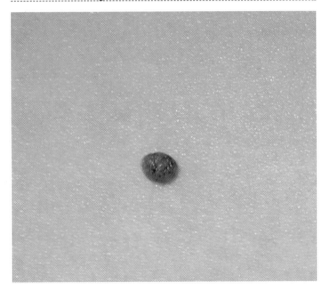

Figure 7-1 • Moles (nevi). *(Image courtesy of Dr. Howard Baden, Massachusetts General Hospital/Harvard Medical School, Boston, MA.)*

■ **Definition**

• Nests of nevus cells (nevomelanocytes) in the epidermis and upper dermis

■ **Etiology**

• The origin of nevus cells is uncertain. They are thought to arise from epidermal melanocytes that descend into the dermis from epidermal melanocytes (nevus cells in the epidermis and upper dermis) and from Schwann cells of nerves (nevus cells in the lower dermis).

■ **Appearance**

- Variety of shapes and sizes.
- Macules (flat), papules (raised, dome shaped), or plaques (raised, flat topped).
- Light brown, dark brown, blue (blue nevus) or skin colored (dermal nevi: melanocytes deep within the dermis).
- May have surrounding halo of depigmentation (halo nevus).
- May be present since birth (congenital nevus) or develop after birth.
- Congenital nevi may be hyperpigmented or have a variety of shades of brown or speckled appearance (nevus spilus).

■ **Diagnosis**

- Biopsy if in doubt; histology shows nevus cells (nevomelanocytes) in grouped clusters (nests).
- Like melanocytes (pigment cells of epidermis), nevomelanocytes lack desmosomes and intercellular attachments.
- Unlike melanocytes, nevomelanocytes are found in nests; melanocytes are usually found singly within the basal layer of the epidermis
- Junctional nevus: nests in epidermis around basement membrane zone.
- Dermal nevus: nests in dermis.
- Compound nevus: nests in both epidermis (around the basement membrane zone) and dermis.

■ **Treatment**

- No need for treatment unless irritated or with significant clinical abnormalities.

Abnormal Moles (Dysplastic Nevi) (Figure 7-2)

■ **Definition**

- Benign neoplasms that have clinical and histologic characteristics sometimes associated with development of melanoma.
- Higher risk for turning into a melanoma than normal mole

■ **Etiology**

- May be genetic component

■ **Appearance**

- Asymmetry
- Border irregularity
- Color variation
- Diameter larger than a pencil eraser
- These are easily remembered as the "ABCD" changes in nevi

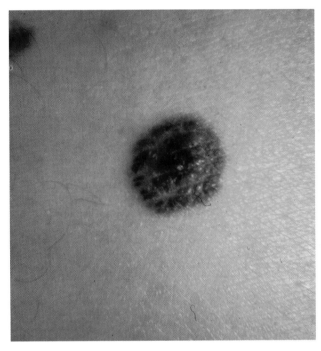

Figure 7-2 • Atypical (dysplastic) nevus. *(Image courtesy of Dr. Howard Baden, Massachusetts General Hospital/Harvard Medical School, Boston, MA.)*

(A for asymmetry, B for border changes, C for color changes, and D for diameter greater than a pencil eraser).

■ **Diagnosis**

- Histopathology: nests (clusters) of melanocytes at the dermo-epidermal junction near the rete ridges of the epidermis, "bridging" of adjacent nests of melanocytes, fibrosis around epidermal rete ridges, and lymphocytic infiltrate in the papillary dermis

■ **Treatment**

- Dermatologists give special attention to atypical nevi, excising those that show significant clinical abnormalities, and carefully following those with fewer clinical abnormalities.
- After a clinically abnormal nevus is excised, if histopathologic examination reveals that the nevus is dysplastic, margins of the specimen removed should be free of atypical cells; if not, reexcision should be performed to remove residual atypical cells

- Persons with a history of dysplastic nevi should be followed at least every 6 months for development of other atypical nevi.
- *Note:* **Dysplastic nevus syndrome (familial atypical nevus syndrome) is seen in families in which many members have large numbers of atypical nevi; members of these families are at increased risk for developing melanoma.**
- A person with multiple atypical nevi and a family history of melanoma has a greatly increased risk for developing melanoma, approaching 100% risk over his or her lifetime.
- Black or otherwise very dark moles, especially on fair-skinned individuals, or moles that are changing can signal development of melanoma and should be examined by a dermatologist.
- Any mole that bleeds or itches should be examined by a dermatologist.
- There is an increased risk for melanoma developing within large congenital nevi (examine regularly and biopsy if any abnormalities).
- A patient should have an examination of his or her moles at least once a year or more frequently if there is a history of abnormal moles or melanoma.

Skin Tags (Acrochordons)

■ **Definition**
- Benign skin growths, usually around the neck or axilla

■ **Etiology**
- Genetic component likely, common in overweight individuals

■ **Appearance**
- Flesh-colored or hyperpigmented, pedunculated (on a stalk) papules

■ **Diagnosis**
- Usually no need for histopathologic examination unless abnormality of growth or doubt as to diagnosis.
- Shave excision and histopathologic examination will then confirm diagnosis.
- Histology: flattened and folded epidermis with dermis of loose connective tissue and dilated blood vessels usually seen around the neck, groin, and axilla, among other locations.

■ **Treatment**
- No need for treatment unless irritated or doubt of diagnosis.
- Irritation: Sometimes irritated by catching on clothing; occasionally pedicle of skin tag will twist, resulting in infarction, pain, and necrosis of skin tag.

- Although suggestions in the literature of possible association between cutaneous skin tags (acrochordons) and adenomatous polyps of the colon, studies to date have not confirmed association.
- For cosmetic or other reasons, skin tags are easily removed by snipping the pedunculated base with sterile scissors, by cryotherapy (using liquid nitrogen), or by electrodessication.
- Patients must be warned that some insurance plans (including Medicare and Medicaid) do not reimburse for removal of skin tags for cosmetic reasons (patient will be charged for procedure).
- Billing Medicare for cosmetic procedures is considered by Medicare to be fraudulent.

Seborrheic Keratoses (Figure 7-3)

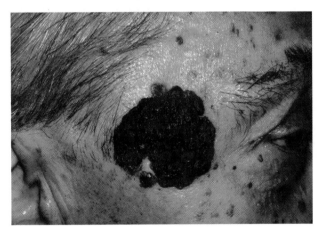

Figure 7-3 • Seborrheic keratoses. *(Image courtesy of Dr. Howard Baden, Massachusetts General Hospital/Harvard Medical School, Boston, MA.)*

■ **Definition**
- Common, benign skin tumors

■ **Etiology**
- No known cause, but appears to be genetic predisposition

■ **Appearance**
- Plaques with hyperpigmentation and hyperkeratosis.
- At first glance may seem to be large moles, but surface rough instead of smooth (mole).
- These "barnacles of life" appear in individuals in their thirties and forties and can be numerous, especially on the back, sides of trunk, abdomen, and under and between breasts.

■ **Diagnosis**
• Biopsy if clinical diagnosis in doubt

■ **Treatment**
• No need for treatment unless growths are irritated or the patient desires treatment for cosmetic reasons; in such case they can be removed by shave excision or treated with liquid nitrogen.

Cutaneous Horn (Figure 7-4)

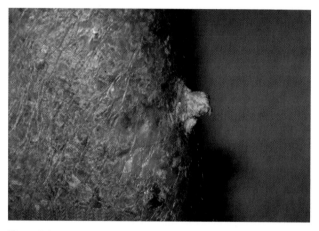

Figure 7-4 • Cutaneous horn. *(Image courtesy of Dr. Howard Baden, Massachusetts General Hospital/Harvard Medical School, Boston, MA.)*

■ **Definition**
• Keratotic lesion that usually appears on the face, arms, or trunk
• Classified as a benign lesion, but can often arise over a squamous cell carcinoma

■ **Etiology**
• Unknown

■ **Appearance**
• Keratotic, horn-shaped lesion protruding from skin

■ **Diagnosis**
• Excise for histology.

■ **Treatment**
• Excise and examine histologically for underlying squamous cell carcinoma.

Keratoacanthoma (Figure 7-5)

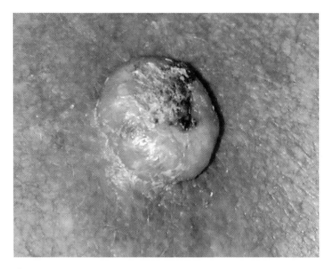

Figure 7-5 · Keratoacanthoma.

■ **Definition**
- Rapidly growing neoplasm usually arising on sun-damaged skin in middle-aged men.
- Often arises over a period of 3 to 6 weeks.
- Females affected half as often as men.
- Usually benign, but with some histologic features of squamous cell carcinoma.
- Unlike squamous cell carcinoma, keratoacanthomas have a tendency to involute.

■ **Etiology**
- Unknown

■ **Appearance**
- Erythematous, dome-shaped nodule with rolled borders and central crust

■ **Diagnosis**
- Biopsy

■ **Treatment**
- Although these lesions have a tendency to involute, it is customary to excise these lesions since they share some histologic features of squamous cell carcinoma.

VASCULAR PROLIFERATIONS AND MALFORMATIONS

- Vascular proliferations can arise from various types of vessels.
- There are many different sizes of such proliferations, from benign vascular proliferations such as tiny telangiectasia (dilation of a tiny vessel), cherry angiomas, and capillary hemangiomas, to large cavernous hemangiomas that affect platelets and circulation.

Hemangioma (Figure 7-6)

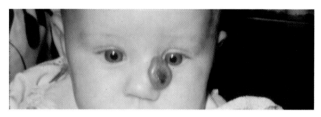

Figure 7-6 • Hemangioma. *(Image courtesy of Dr. Howard Baden, Massachusetts General Hospital/Harvard Medical School, Boston, MA.)*

■ Definition
- Benign proliferation of blood vessels.
- Some hemangiomas consist of arterial proliferations; some consist of venular proliferations.
- Some tend to spontaneously regress (capillary hemangiomas).
- Some show little tendency to involute (cavernous hemangiomas).

■ Etiology
- Unknown

■ Appearance
- Capillary hemangiomas: blood vessels at the end branches of the arterial system, each lined by a single endothelial cell
- Cavernous hemangiomas: composed of venular structures

■ Diagnosis
- Cavernous hemangiomas: check platelets and hemoglobin.

■ Treatment
- Lasers may be useful to ablate vascular lesions where necessary.
- Systemic corticosteroids can be helpful in shrinking hemangiomas that impinge on vital structures.

Port-Wine Stain (Figure 7-7)

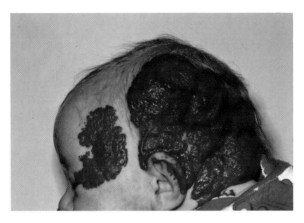

Figure 7-7 • Port-wine stain. *(Image courtesy of Dr. Howard Baden, Massachusetts General Hospital/Harvard Medical School, Boston, MA.)*

■ **Definition**
- Vascular malformation of the upper dermis, usually on the face or neck

■ **Etiology**
- Thought to originate from developmental defect in embryogenesis during the time that the vascular system is developing

■ **Appearance**
- Pink patch at birth; during adulthood these lesions darken to a purple color and sometimes develop a rough surface.

■ **Diagnosis**
- Diagnosis by clinical appearance and history.
- Large port-wine stains on the face should prompt investigation of potential underlying ophthalmologic or neurologic disorders.
- Patients with involvement in the area of the first branch of the trigeminal nerve should be evaluated for glaucoma.

■ **Treatment**
- Treatment with pulsed-dye laser may improve appearance.

Venous Lake

■ **Definition**
- Purplish blue papules often found on lips of older patients

■ **Etiology**
- Caused by loss of elasticity of vessel walls, causing dilation of the vessels.
- Damage from long exposure to ultraviolet radiation can cause these lesions.

■ **Appearance**
- Purplish blue, soft papules on lips

■ **Diagnosis**
- None; biopsy if in doubt of diagnosis

■ **Treatment**
- No need for treatment

Cherry Angioma

■ **Definition**
- Common neoplasms found on the trunk and sometimes on the face

■ **Etiology**
- Unknown; probably genetic factor

■ **Appearance**
- Appear in adulthood clinically as small red/purple papules on the trunk and sometimes on the face
- Usually increase in number during adulthood

■ **Diagnosis**
- Biopsy if in doubt
- Histology: numerous dilated venules and collagenous stroma

■ **Treatment**
- No need for treatment unless the lesions bleed or are irritated.
- Patients may desire treatment for cosmetic reasons.
- Lesions can be removed by electrodessication or by excision.

Pyogenic Granuloma (Figure 7-8)

■ **Definition**
- Bleeding papule

■ **Etiology**
- No known precipitating cause for the origination of a pyogenic granuloma, but sometimes occurs during pregnancy or after minor trauma to an area

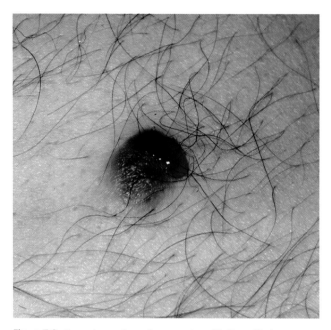

Figure 7-8 • Pyogenic granuloma. *(Image courtesy of Dr. Howard Baden, Massachusetts General Hospital/Harvard Medical School, Boston, MA.)*

■ **Appearance**
- Pink papule; patient usually presents with a bandage over the lesion because it continues to bleed.

■ **Diagnosis**
- Histology: proliferation of capillaries or venules

■ **Treatment**
- Shave excision followed by electrodessication of the base of the lesion

Telangiectasia

■ **Definition**
- Tiny blood vessels near skin surface

■ **Etiology**
- May occur from sun damage, from estrogen effects (during pregnancy or while taking oral contraceptives or hormone replacement), or from liver cirrhosis.

■ **Appearance**
• Spiderlike, tiny blood vessels

■ **Diagnosis**
• Clinical appearance

■ **Treatment**
• For troublesome lesions on face: Treatment with electrodessi-cation (electrocautery with a fine needle) or laser can be effective.
• Telangiectasia on legs: hypertonic saline leg vein injections by an expert.

MALIGNANT GROWTHS (SKIN CANCERS)

Melanoma (Figure 7-9)

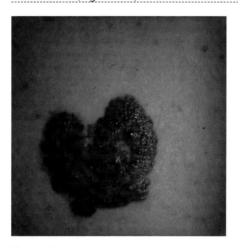

Figure 7-9 • Melanoma. *(Image courtesy of Dr. Howard Baden, Massachusetts General Hospital/Harvard Medical School, Boston, MA.)*

■ **Definition**
• Malignant proliferation of melanocytes (pigment cells)
• Potentially the most deadly of skin cancers

■ **Etiology**
• Can arise from a mole or may arise *de novo* and can metasta-size and invade any organ.
• There is greater risk for melanoma developing in atypical nevi than in normal nevi.

- Appears to be a hereditary factor involved in development of melanomas.
- Melanomas can arise sporadically, however, without any family history of melanoma.
- Sunlight appears to play a role in the etiology of melanoma, especially intermittent exposure in the early years and blistering sunburns in childhood.

■ Appearance

- Macules, papules, plaques, nodules, or other shapes
- Usually intensely hyperpigmented or with variegated color, rarely amelanotic (without pigmentation)
- Often asymmetric, with irregular borders, and with variation in color such as mixture of black and browns (these are also clinical characteristics of atypical nevi)
- *Note:* Danger signs in moles

   A: asymmetry
   B: border irregularity
   C: color changes
   D: diameter greater in size than a pencil eraser

■ Diagnosis

- Chest x-ray should be obtained for any patient with a melanoma that invades the dermis.
- Sentinal node biopsy helpful for prognosis of melanomas greater than 1.0 mm and less than 4.0 mm in depth.
- Further treatment such as lymph node dissection may be performed based on results of sentinal node biopsy.

■ Treatment

- Lesions suspicious for melanoma should be excised; if melanoma is diagnosed, wide reexcision of excision site should be performed.
- Reexcision of margins (excision of normal skin surrounding the melanoma):
  - Melanomas up to 1 mm in thickness: 1 cm reexcision margins
  - Melanomas greater than 1 mm in thickness: 2 cm margins
- *In situ* (melanoma cells confined to epidermis) lesions should be dissected down into the subcutaneous fat.
- In all other lesions, subcutaneous fat should be removed down to fascia.
- Chemotherapy or immunotherapy are adjuvant therapies for advanced stages of melanoma, but no satisfactory results that extend survival have yet been obtained.
- Regular follow-up every 6 months necessary after excision of melanoma.

- Nodes should always be palpated for enlargement at the time of detection of melanoma and in subsequent examinations.
- *Note:* Excision of *in situ* melanoma carries an excellent prognosis. Once the dermis has been invaded by melanoma cells, the prognosis becomes less favorable, depending on the depth of invasion and any metastasis. See Appendix B for staging of melanomas and prognosis.

Basal Cell Carcinoma (Figure 7-10)

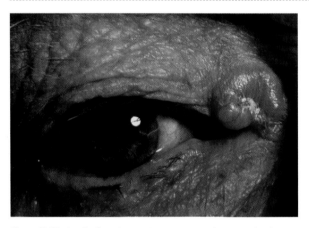

Figure 7-10 • Basal cell carcinoma. *(Image courtesy of Dr. Howard Baden, Massachusetts General Hospital/Harvard Medical School, Boston, MA.)*

■ Definition
- Basal cell carcinoma is the most common skin cancer and is found in middle-aged adults.

■ Etiology
- Sun exposure increases the risk for developing basal cell carcinoma.

■ Appearance
- Usually a pink, pearly papule or nodule with rolled borders and telangiectasia coursing over its surface
- Commonly found on face, ears, upper chest, or upper back
- Often with ulcerated center
- Can also appear as a pink waxy plaque, an atrophic, white waxy plaque, or a huge, ulcerated tumor
- At an early stage, may appear as a slightly pink papule with pearl-like sheen

■ **Diagnosis**

- Any new, erythematous papule that persists should be checked by a dermatologist.
- Lesions suspicious for basal cell carcinoma should be examined via biopsy.
- Histopathology: basal cells with numerous mitotic figures, proliferating down into dermis.

■ **Treatment**

- Excision with margins satisfactory to remove all residual carcinomatous basal cells.
- Patients with a history of basal cell carcinoma should be checked every 6 months for recurrences or development of new lesions.
- Mohs' surgery is very useful for excising basal cell carcinomas on the face, where margins must be clear but as much tissue as possible needs to be preserved.
- Mohs' surgeons: dermatologists who have obtained additional training to perform step-wise excisions and processing to maximize all tumor cell removal and minimize normal tissue removed.
- Clinical trials are in progress to test effectiveness of immunotherapy of some basal cell carcinoma.
- Although basal cell carcinoma rarely metastasizes, the tumor can erode down into underlying bone and tissue and result in grotesque disfigurement.
- *Note:* **A genetic defect is the cause of the basal cell nevus syndrome, a condition characterized by numerous basal cell carcinomas that develop over a patient's lifetime.**

Squamous Cell Carcinoma (Figure 7-11)

■ **Definition**

- Second most common skin cancer; most commonly found in the elderly
- Often found at the base of the cutaneous horn (keratotic skin projection)
- Sometimes found at the base of a keratoacanthoma (lesion resembling basal cell carcinoma)
- May develop in some actinic keratoses over time

■ **Etiology**

- Sun exposure increases the risk for developing squamous cell carcinoma.
- Bowen's disease is a superficial squamous cell carcinoma (pink, scaly patch) often found in non-sun-exposed area

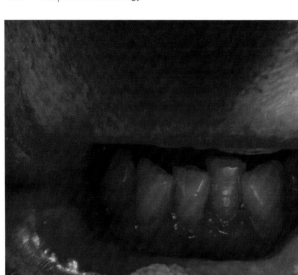

Figure 7-11 • Squamous cell carcinoma. *(Image courtesy of Dr. Howard Baden, Massachusetts General Hospital/Harvard Medical School, Boston, MA.)*

■ Appearance

- Variable in appearance but usually nodules or plaques in sun-exposed areas with erythema, scale, and hyperkeratosis.
- Wart-like projections on the face, ears, scalp, or anterior lower legs are particularly suspicious for squamous cell carcinoma.

■ Diagnosis

- Biopsy, histology: proliferation of atypical squamous cells extending into the dermis, frequent mitotic figures, varying degrees of differentiation of the cells, "squamous eddies" and "horn pearls" (swirl-like arrangements of epidermal cells), acantholysis, intraepithelial abscesses

■ Treatment

- Excision with margins cleared of any residual tumor cells.
- Although rarely metastasizing unless large, squamous cell carcinoma has more potential for metastasis than basal cell carcinoma.

- A particularly aggressive form of squamous cell carcinoma with greater potential for metastasis is basosquamous cell carcinoma, with features of both squamous cell and basal cell carcinoma.
- Persons with a history of squamous cell carcinoma should be checked every 6 months for recurrences or development of new lesions.
- Very superficial squamous cell carcinoma (Bowen's disease) may respond to fluorouracil cream (Efudex) bid for 3 to 4 weeks.

Merkel's Cell Carcinoma

■ Definition
- Uncommon cutaneous neuroendocrine carcinoma associated with Merkel's cells (touch receptors found around hair follicles and in the basal layer of skin).
- Tumors highly invasive, poor prognosis.
- Often associated with squamous cell carcinoma or other neoplasms.
- Distant metastases, most commonly to lymph nodes, liver, bone, brain, lung, and skin, occur in approximately half of patients.
- Death is usual result of distant metastases.

■ Etiology
- Unknown

■ Appearance
- Painless, pink or red nodules, sometimes with ulceration
- Most commonly found on head or neck
- Usually in the sixth or seventh decade of life
- Occur with equal frequency in men and women

■ Diagnosis
- Immunocytochemistry helpful in differentiating Merkel's cell carcinoma from other tumors.
- Dense core granules characteristically found in cells of Merkel's cell carcinoma.
- Electron microscopy useful for confirming dense core granules.
- Microscopic features of Merkel's cell carcinoma similar to those of metastatic oat cell carcinoma; radiologic studies of the lung should be conducted to rule out oat cell carcinoma.

■ Treatment
- Excise Merkel's cell tumors with wide margins, followed by radiation and/or chemotherapy.
- Regional lymph node dissection often necessary.

Kaposi's Sarcoma

■ **Definition**

- Vascular neoplasm originally described in elderly men of Mediterranean origin and Jewish descent.
- Affects skin and subcutaneous tissue and can infiltrate the lung, causing shortness of breath, and the gastrointestinal tract, causing intestinal bleeding.
- Liver, spleen, and lymph nodes may be involved.
- An aggressive form of Kaposi's sarcoma is found in patients with AIDS, most commonly in homosexual men.

■ **Etiology**

- AIDS-associated Kaposi's sarcoma has been found to be associated with HHV-8 (sometimes called Kaposi's sarcoma–associated herpesvirus, although a direct role in the development of Kaposi's sarcoma has not been established).
- Further studies will be necessary to determine whether prophylaxis against HHV-8 infection will decrease the incidence of development of AIDS-associated Kaposi's sarcoma.

■ **Appearance**

- Firm, reddish brown, purple, pink, or bluish macules, papules, plaques, or nodules that may ulcerate

■ **Diagnosis**

- Histology: abnormal vascularization, proliferating endothelial cells and fibroblasts, and spindle-shaped tumor cells

■ **Treatment**

- Antiretroviral drugs, chemotherapy, interferons, radiation
- Early in development, lesions can be treated with liquid nitrogen cryotherapy, photodynamic therapy, intralesional chemotherapy, radiation, and topical retinoids.

LYMPHOMAS AND LEUKEMIAS

Lymphomas and leukemias can directly infiltrate the skin, such as in leukemia cutis or cutaneous B-cell and T-cell lymphomas, or the skin can react to internal, systemic problems associated with lymphomas and leukemias without direct infiltration of the skin with the abnormal cells.

Leukemia Cutis

■ **Definition**

- Infiltration and proliferation of leukemia cells into skin that can occur in patients with leukemia

■ **Etiology**
• Leukemia

■ **Appearance**
• Chronic lymphocytic leukemia: tumors and nodules on head, neck, and trunk; plaques with erythema on hands
• Myelogenous leukemia: skin changes similar but occur less frequently than in lymphocytic leukemia
• Adult T-cell leukemia: maculopapular rash, erythroderma, nodules, bullous lesions

■ **Diagnosis**
• Biopsy with histochemical and immunohistochemical studies

■ **Treatment**
• Treatment of underlying leukemia with radiotherapy and chemotherapy.
• Whole-body electron beam radiation to skin may be helpful.

Cutaneous T-Cell Lymphoma (CTCL) (Mycosis Fungoides)

■ **Definition**
• Group of entities characterized by proliferation of T-lymphocytes in skin

■ **Etiology**
• Unknown

■ **Appearance**
• Patch stage (early): patches of erythema and scale on skin, history of "chronic dermatitis," may last for years; eventually evolves into plaque stage
• Plaque stage: plaques with erythema and scale; can eventually develop into tumor stage
• Tumor stage (late, more aggressive phase); ulcerated red-brown nodules over the body. Sézary's syndrome occurs when large numbers of CTCL cells circulate in the blood, causing erythroderma (red skin)

■ **Diagnosis**
• Biopsy may not be diagnostic in early patch stage
• Eventually biopsy will show diagnostic signs of hyperchromatic, hyperconvuluted lymphocytes, some forming Pautrier's microabscesses (clusters of lymphocytes surrounded by a clear space), and epidermotrophism (tendency to migrate into the epidermis).

- Immunohistochemical studies can identify types of malignant T cells in tissue and blood.
- Staging is done on the basis of type of skin involvement, lymph node involvement, peripheral blood involvement, and visceral organ involvement. Prognosis and therapy depend on the particular stage involved.

■ **Treatment**

- PUVA, topical nitrogen mustard therapy, methotrexate, radiotherapy, total skin radiotherapy, and interferon-alpha.
- Patients in patch stage can be kept under reasonable control, usually for many years, with topical corticosteroids or topical nitrogen mustard (topical nitrogen mustard is toxic to lymphocytes).
- There is no cure when the disease progresses into the tumor stage.

Cutaneous B-Cell Lymphoma

■ **Definition**

- Skin manifestations of B-cell lymphoma

■ **Etiology**

- Unknown

■ **Appearance**

- Deep red, smooth nodules in skin, especially on head and neck.
- There are different types of B-cell lymphoma, both large cell and small cell.

■ **Diagnosis**

- Biopsy and immunohistochemical evaluation will be helpful in determining type and prognosis.

■ **Treatment**

- Surgical excision is sometimes effective if lesions are few and localized.
- Systemic therapy may be required with chemotherapy, systemic steroids, retinoids, or interferon.

Sweet's Syndrome (Acute Febrile Neutrophilic Dermatosis) (Figure 7-12)

■ **Definition**

- There are general reactive phenomena to leukemias and lymphomas, including fever, pruritus, purpura, bruising, and sometimes

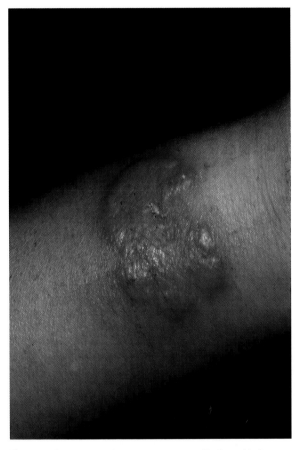

Figure 7-12 • Sweet's syndrome. *(Image courtesy of Dr. Howard Baden, Massachusetts General Hospital/Harvard Medical School, Boston, MA.)*

erythroderma or ichthyosis. There are also more specific, reactive, paraneoplastic phenomena to hematopoietic malignancies, such as Sweet's syndrome.
- Most frequently associated with acute myelogenous leukemia.
- Occasionally Sweet's syndrome is found in association with malignancies associated with the genitourinary tract or (less frequently) the respiratory tract.

■ **Etiology**
- Unknown

■ **Appearance**

- Tender, violaceous nodules and plaques, especially on the dorsal aspects of the hands
- Fever and peripheral neutrophilia, elevated sedimentation rate and leukocytosis, ANCA
- *Note: ANCA frequently found in Wegener's granulomatosis.*

■ **Diagnosis**

- Histology: spongiosis with intraepidermal vesicle formation and degeneration of the reticular dermis as well as prominent infiltration of the dermis with neutrophils.
- Unlike leukemia cutis, there are no leukemia cells in the lesions.

■ **Treatment**

- Systemic corticosteroids (0.5–1.0 mg/kg per day), dapsone (100–200 mg per day), potassium iodide (900 mg per day), or colchicine (1.5 mg per day)

Erythroderma

■ **Definition**

- Reactive process that can occur with T-cell leukemia and lymphoma

■ **Etiology**

- The cause of erythroderma is either unknown or secondary to a wide variety of disorders that include underlying malignancies, such as mycosis fungoides; psoriasis, drug reaction, collagen vascular disease, and ichthyosis

■ **Appearance**

- Redness of skin, accompanied by (or followed by) exfoliation

■ **Diagnosis**

- Erythroderma is a serious condition; the underlying cause should be quickly sought.
- Histology: may be nonspecific with vascular ectasia and infiltration with lymphocytes or may be specific for underlying conditions such as ichthyosis or psoriasis.

■ **Treatment**

- Treatment of underlying cause, maintaining electrolyte and fluid balance, monitoring for sepsis.
- Topical steroids and emollients helpful.
- If underlying cause of erythroderma is not known, search for underlying malignancy.

Ichthyosis (Figure 7-13)

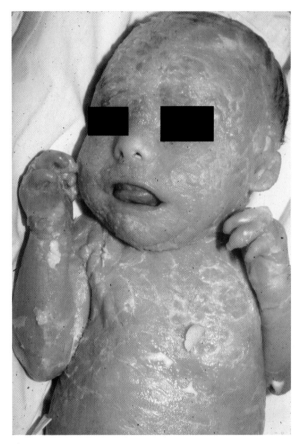

Figure 7-13 • Lamellar ichthyosis. *(Image courtesy of Dr. Howard Baden, Massachusetts General Hospital/Harvard Medical School, Boston, MA.)*

■ **Definition**
- Dry, sometimes erythematous skin

■ **Etiology**
- Inherited or acquired
- Acquired ichthyosis can be paraneoplastic and occur prior to or simultaneously with Hodgkin's lymphoma, non-Hodgkin's lymphoma, and mycosis fungoides.
- Ichthyosis can also signal myeloma, cancer of the breast or cervix, cancer of the lung, or other malignancies.

■ **Appearance**
- Dry, hyperkeratotic skin

■ **Diagnosis**
- Biopsy if diagnosis in doubt.
- Clinical appearance can suggest type if inherited.

■ **Treatment**
- Treatment of the underlying problem if possible
- Topical corticosteroids if inflammation is present
- Skin emollients for dryness

What to Tell Your Patients about Skin Care

For routine cleansing of skin and body, a mild, unscented soap should be used. Good basic soaps and moisturizers can be obtained over the counter in the drug store.

Dry Skin

For dry skin, an unscented moisturizer should be applied. It is especially important to apply moisturizer within the first minute or two of toweling dry after bathing to prevent evaporation of moisturizer from skin. Moisturizer should also be applied to hands after each washing. Dry heat in the winter worsens dry skin; a humidifier added to a room or to the house heating system can lessen the drying effect.

Sun Protection

Sunscreen should always be applied for sun protection, even if outside for only a brief period of time and even on a cloudy day or in winter on the ski slopes. Sunscreen that protects against both UVA and UVB is best; SPF 15 is usually sufficient for normal activities with only occasional sun exposure. When going on a walk or in the sun for more than occasional exposure, SPF in the thirties or forties should be used. Sunscreen should be reapplied after swimming or if perspiring, since it will wash off, whether promoted as "water-proof" or not. Sun-protective clothing should also be used as extra protection. A hat should be worn to protect a bald head or a head with thinning hair.

Skin Aging

There are two types of skin aging: intrinsic ("internal time clock") and extrinsic (caused by the environment). There is no way yet to prevent intrinsic aging, but extrinsic aging (photoaging) can be prevented. The sun ages skin. Most wrinkles and mottled pigmentation are due to sun damage; therefore, sunscreen is important. Tretinoin (Renova) is an FDA-approved, prescription product for treatment of fine (not deep) wrinkles. The best treatment available now against skin aging is prevention of sun damage.

Loss of Hair

There are many potential causes of loss of hair (alopecia). Scalp conditions can contribute to hair loss. There are also natural reasons for hair loss. Hair goes through natural "resting" (telogen) cycles and during these times hair may appear not as thick. Androgenic alopecia is caused by hereditary factors and aging. Stress (childbirth, surgeries) can precipitate *telogen effluvium* (loss of resting hairs). Medications and illness can precipitate hair loss, including *anagen effluvium* (loss of growing hairs). Thyroid dysfunction or hormone changes can precipitate hair loss (check thyroid function and testosterone levels). Alopecia areata, characterized by loss of hair in rounded patches, is caused by lymphocyte autoimmune attack upon hair follicles. Many other disease processes affect hair growth. To minimize hair loss from trauma to hair, gentle treatment is important. Hair should not be combed when wet or curled, twisted, or pulled back into a pony tail. A medicated shampoo is helpful for scalp itching or scaling. Tinea capitis (fungal infection) should be suspected in children with loss of hair and scaling of scalp; examine scalp scrapings and pulled hairs under the microscope for hyphae.

Unwanted Hair

Unwanted hair can be treated with electrolysis, wax epilation, bleaching, shaving, or laser treatment. Skin irritation can result, however, from such treatment. Electrolysis and laser hair removal can permanently destroy unwanted hair if the dermal papilla of the hair follicle is destroyed, but many treatments are usually necessary.

Itching (Pruritus)

Itching is common in the elderly. It can be precipitated in all age groups by a variety of causes. Medications can precipate itching. Certain medications are more likely than others to cause itching: check the *Physicians Desk Reference* for side effects of medications. Fragrances can cause itching, and they are present in many soaps, moisturizers, hairsprays, cosmetics, and bath powders, and in all perfumes. Hepatic or renal dysfunction and underlying malignancies or other disorders can precipitate itching. AIDS can precipitate itching. Certain fabrics (or certain dyes in fabrics) can precipitate itching. Dry skin can precipitate itching. A mild, unscented soap is important for bathing. An unscented moisturizer after bathing offsets dry skin. Topical Sarna lotion (contains menthol) can be useful for localized itching, and oral antihistamine is helpful for more severe itching.

A

Opportunities in Dermatology

Dermatology is a very nice specialty. Hours can be tailored to the physician's needs, there are not many emergencies, and call schedules are not usually onerous. Patients can be helped in important ways. Irritating and disfiguring skin problems can usually be treated, and the patient's morale and self-esteem are lifted with improved appearance. Diagnosis can be fun. Behind each patient examination door is a patient with a skin problem and clues waiting to be put together.

Dermatology visits are shorter than those in some other specialities. Because the visits are usually relatively short, there may be 20 to 25 patients or more scheduled in a morning or afternoon clinical session. The most likely diagnosis for each patient is determined, as is whether further diagnostic procedures are necessary. A treatment plan is developed and executed. The dermatologist discusses with the patient the particular problem and treatment as well as elements in good skin care and importance of sun protection. The dermatologist must understand the structure and functions of skin, what goes wrong to result in disease, and what the skin looks like in those diseases. It is also important to understand the entire body to understand dermatologic disorders. Skin is the largest organ of the body and often reflects the condition of the underlying body. For those interested in research, skin is the ideal organ for study. It is easily accessible and is an excellent system for both clinical and basic research.

Dermatology residency programs vary, but in general they are 3 years in duration. In a few academic programs, a year of research may be added. During the 3 years, the resident learns how to examine a problem, create a good differential of possible diagnoses, and put together clues from the patient's history, subjective symptoms, and objective findings. The resident will participate in patient care, often in a variety of clinical settings in affiliation with the academic center. There may be, for example, clinical rotations in an affiliated Veterans Administration hospital dermatology clinic, in a public health clinic for sexually transmitted diseases and in the dermatology clinics within the primary academic center. The dermatology resident will learn how to excise nevi, cysts, skin cancers, and other lesions and may learn some cosmetic procedures involving laser treatment, liposuction, autologous fat transfer, tissue augmentation, and chemical peels.

Because dermatology is a popular speciality, dermatology residency slots are very competitive. There are many applicants and only a few slots. For those interested in applying to a dermatology residency program, it is important to express interest early to dermatology faculty members and residents, gain their advice about how to enhance chances of securing a dermatology residency, and actively participate in a dermatology rotation. This should be done both in the dermatology department in the academic institution where the medical student has trained as well as in any other locations where the student is interested in entering into dermatology residency. References from the "home academic institution" are valuable in securing a residency, and demonstrating true interest and enthusiasm in the training institution as well as in other potential institutions is vital.

Selection of residents is usually by the dermatology faculty plus either a resident delegate or other form of input from the residents. The residency selection committee will be looking for good grades during medical school, good board scores, exceptional performance in the dermatology rotation, and evidence of drive and enthusiasm for becoming a dermatologist. Enthusiasm for dermatology is demonstrated by active participation in a dermatology rotation with a good base of knowledge and participation in events within the dermatology department, such as "Journal Club" and "Grand Rounds," that increase knowledge and exposure to dermatology. The committee wants people that are congenial, cheerful, helpful, hardworking, studious, liked by the residents, and sensitive to patients' problems and needs. For those interested in research, web sites of many academic institutions lead to information about ongoing research at that institution in cutaneous (skin) biology. Inquiries about research opportunities can be made to the individual scientists conducting research in areas of the student's interest, by letter or email, with enclosed résumé. Research experience is often an excellent demonstration to the dermatology residency committee of interest and enthusiasm for dermatology. For more information about dermatology residency programs, see the web site of the American Academy of Dermatology at *www.aad.org.*

B Review Questions and Answers

QUESTIONS

Multiple Choice

Choose the single best answer.

1. The basement membrane
   A. separates the dermis from the epidermis.
   B. separates the dermis from the subcutaneous fat.
   C. is composed of a layer of cells called the basal layer.
   D. is found at the bottom of each cell in the cornified layer of skin.
   E. is composed primarily of elastic fibers.

2. Melanocytes
   A. are pigment-producing cells normally found in the dermis.
   B. transfer melanin to fibroblasts through tiny packets called melanophores.
   C. In dark skin, melanin is gathered together in membrane-bound groups of melanosomes.
   D. Ultraviolet light destroys melanocytes, releasing melanin granules produced by the melanocytes.
   E. transfer melanosomes to the lower layers of the epidermis.

3. Dendritic cells that play an important immune function of the epidermis
   A. T-lymphocytes
   B. B-lymphocytes
   C. Langerhan's cells
   D. Merkel's cells
   E. fibroblasts

4. The growth phase of the hair cycle is called
   A. catagen.
   B. telogen.
   C. anagen.
   D. papillary phase.
   E. dermal papilla.

5. "Moth-eaten alopecia" is characteristic of
   A. syphilis.
   B. alopecia areata.
   C. alopecia universalis.
   D. lice infestation.
   E. moth egg infestation.

6. Latex allergy is

   A. a result of contact with Musk ambrette and Parsol.
   B. due to thiazides and furocoumarins.
   C. an example of contact urticaria.
   D. manifested as a rash over the knuckles of the hand.
   E. self-limited and of little consequence.

7. Allergic contact dermatitis is

   A. an IgE-mediated, immediate hypersensitivity response.
   B. a delayed-hypersensitivity, cell-mediated immune response, type IV.
   C. an irritant contact dermatitis.
   D. an immunologic reaction involving B-cell pathways, with immediate clinical manifestations.
   E. none of the above.

8. White piedra is caused by

   A. *Piedraia hortae.*
   B. *Trichosporon beigelii.*
   C. *Malassezia furfur.*
   D. *Exophiala werneckii.*
   E. *Phaeoannellomyces werneckii.*

9. Chancroid is caused by

   A. *Phaeoannellomyces werneckii (Exophiala werneckii).*
   B. papillomavirus.
   C. poxvirus.
   D. *Haemophilus ducreyi.*
   E. herpesvirus.

10. Pediculus humanus corporis is

    A. another name for skin tags.
    B. a toenail fungus.
    C. a body louse.
    D. a mite.
    E. a bacteria.

11. Scabies

    A. can remain dormant within the trigeminal nerve root ganglion.
    B. is caused by mites that burrow into skin and lay eggs.
    C. is an infection with yellow crusting of skin.
    D. is caused by fleas.
    E. is caused by ticks.

12. Erythema infectiosum ("fifth disease" or "slapped cheeks") is caused by

    A. *Streptococcus* group A.
    B. poxvirus.
    C. varicella zoster virus.
    D. HPV.
    E. parvovirus B19.

13. Scarlet fever

    A. is caused by circulating toxin produced by *Staphylococcus aureus*.
    B. "White-strawberry" tongue may be present.
    C. Litia's lines may be present.
    D. is characterized by a vesicular rash on trunk and extremities.
    E. usually occurs in adults.

14. Syphilis

    A. is often called "the great imitator."
    B. Primary lesion is a painful chancre.
    C. is caused by coronavirus.
    D. is often associated with alopecia areata.
    E. Primary lesion is a diffuse rash.

15. Rocky Mountain spotted fever

    A. is caused by *Rickettsia prowazekii*.
    B. Rash begins on the trunk and spreads to wrists, hands, and ankles.
    C. is a dangerous infection that must be recognized and treated.
    D. There is no treatment for this disorder.
    E. There is no need for treatment for this disorder.

16. Kawasaki's disease

    A. is an acute, vascular disease of unknown origin that occurs during childhood.
    B. "Cherry red lips" and "strawberry tongue."
    C. Fever is followed by a morbilliform eruption.
    D. Coronary artery aneurysms can occur.
    E. All of the above.

17. Atopic dermatitis

    A. is a chronic disorder usually beginning in late adulthood.
    B. is often associated with a history of malnutrition.
    C. is nonpruritic.
    D. Superimposed infection often occurs.
    E. All of the above.

18. Toxic epidermal necrolysis

    A. is a self-limited disorder resulting in rash from environmental toxins.
    B. Skin of fingers becomes "bound down" and sclerotic.
    C. is an allergic contact reaction.
    D. Fluid retention in skin leads to edema.
    E. Severe end of spectrum of hypersensitivity reactions.

19. Pruritic urticarial papules of pregnancy

    A. is a pruritic eruption of erythematous vesicles.
    B. typically develops during the first trimester of pregnancy.
    C. is caused by herpesvirus 8.
    D. Rash will usually resolve after delivery of the baby.
    E. is characterized by nonpruritic papules that typically develop in the third trimester of pregnancy.

20. Herpes gestationis
    A. is caused by the herpesvirus.
    B. is annular or serpentiginous lesions composed of bullae or vesicles that extend over the abdomen, to other parts of the trunk, and to extremities.
    C. is nonpruritic.
    D. poses significant risk to the fetus.
    E. All of the above.

Matching

21. Choose the best match:

    1. *Pityrosporum ovale* may play a role.
    2. New lesions arise at the site of trauma to normal skin.
    3. Plaques with erythema, lichenification
    4. Sebaceous glands stimulated by circulating androgens precipitate this condition.
    5. Extension of blister by applying pressure.
    6. Follicular occlusion of apocrine ducts.
    7. Often occurs after bathing in hot tubs.

    A. Lichen simplex chronicus
    B. Folliculitis
    C. Hidradenitis suppurativa and scale
    D. Koebner's phenomennon
    E. Seborrheic dermatitis
    F. Nikolsky's sign
    G. Acne

22. Match the correct term for the corresponding skin condition:

    1. Skin dryness
    2. Cracking
    3. Itching
    4. Redness

    A. Pruritus
    B. Xerosis
    C. Erythema
    D. Fissuring

23. Match the condition with the associated malignancy:

    1. Sweet's syndrome
    2. Subcutaneous fat necrosis
    3. Dermatomyositis

    A. Benign condition associated with obesity or marker for malignancies, especially gastric adenocarcinoma
    B. Carcinoma of esophagus, stomach, bladder, prostate, breast, lung, or cervix
    C. Acinar cell adenocarcinoma of pancreas, pancreatitis, or pancreatic pseudocyst

4. Acanthosis nigricans

5. Erythema gyratum repens

6. Necrolytic migratory erythema

7. Paraneoplastic acrokeratosis of Bazex

D. Glucagonoma

E. Cancer of upper respiratory tract

F. Myelocytic leukemia

G. Bronchogenic carcinoma or cancer of breast, ovary, or cervix

24. Match the following conditions with associated abnormalities:

1. Basal cell nevus syndrome

2. Xeroderma pigmentosum

3. Porphyria

4. Pseudoxanthoma elasticum

5. Ehlers-Danlos syndrome

6. Incontinentia pigmenti

7. Ectodermal dysplasias

8. Ichthyoses

A. Abnormalities of connective tissue, "cobblestone" appearance of skin

B. Whorled slate-gray macular pigmentation

C. Defects in repair of damage from ultraviolet radiation with development of skin cancers

D. Hyperelastic skin, poor wound healing

E. Affects the cornified layer of skin

F. Deficiency in the heme biosynthesis pathway, photosensitivity

G. Abnormal development of hair, teeth, nails, sweat glands, skin, eyes, and ears

H. Basal cell carcinomas and jaw cysts

25. Match the following types of fungal infections:

1. Hair

2. Nails

3. Hands

4. Feet

5. Groin

6. Face

7. Beard area of face

8. Skin

A. Tinea pedis

B. Tinea facei

C. Tinea capitis

D. Tinea corporis

E. Tinea manus

F. Onychomycosis

G. Tinea barbae

H. Tinea cruris

ANSWER KEY

1. A	11. B	21. 1E, 2D, 3A, 4G, 5F, 6C, 7B
2. E	12. E	22. 1B, 2D, 3A, 4C
3. C	13. B	23. 1F, 2C, 3G, 4A, 5B, 6D, 7E
4. C	14. A	
5. A	15. C	24. 1H, 2C, 3F, 4A, 5D, 6B, 7G, 8E
6. C	16. E	
7. B	17. D	25. 1C, 2F, 3E, 4A, 5H, 6B, 7G, 8D
8. B	18. E	
9. D	19. D	
10. C	20. B	

ANSWERS

1. **A. The basement membrane separates the dermis from the epidermis.** The epidermis, not the basement membrane, is composed of a layer of cells called the basal layer. The basal layer of cells is found in the lower epidermis abutting the basement membrane. Type IV collagen is a major component of the basement membrane.

2. **E. Melanocytes are pigment-producing cells normally found in the epidermis that transfer melanosomes to the lower layers of the epidermis through tiny packets called melanophores.** Fibroblasts reside in the dermis and do not normally receive pigment. In light skin, melanin is gathered together in membrane-bound groups of melanosomes. In dark skin, the melanosomes are dispersed individually throughout the cytoplasm of keratinocytes. Melanocytes proliferate in response to ultraviolet light or inflammatory processes and produce melanin in packets called melanosomes.

3. **C. *Langerhan's cells* are dendritic cells in the epidermis that play an important immune function in skin by detecting antigen, processing the antigen, presenting it to the T cells, and activating the T cells.** *Merkel's cells* are slow-adapting touch receptors in the epidermis to which unmyelinated, free nerve endings associate. T-lymphocytes and B-lymphocytes are not dendritic cells. Fibroblasts are found in the dermis, not the epidermis.

4. **C. Anagen is the growth phase of the hair cycle.** Telogen is the resting phase of the hair cycle. Catagen is the involutional phase of the hair cycle. The dermal papilla at the base of the hair follicle plays an important role in stimulating anagen.

5. **A. Syphilis is often associated with hair loss with a "moth-eaten" appearance.** Loss of hair of the entire scalp is characteristic of alopecia totalis. Alopecia universalis is loss of hair on the entire body.

6. **C. Latex allergy can result in contact urticaria, an IgE-mediated, immediate hypersensitivity response.** There may be immediate development of urticaria (hives) with swelling of face, lips, and mucosa. Anaphylactic reaction can occasionally result. Contact with *latex* can result in a medical emergency with the need for immediate treatment with antihistamines, epinephrine, and corticosteroids. Musk ambrette (in perfumes) and Parsol (in some sunscreens) are photoallergans; thiazides and furocoumarins are phototoxic substances.

7. **B. Allergic contact dermatitis is a delayed-hypersensitivity, cell-mediated immune response, type IV.** Contact urticaria is an IgE-mediated, immediate-hypersensitivity response. Most people develop irritant contact dermatitis immediately following contact with an irritating substance (e.g., lye or ammonia). Allergic contact dermatitis is an immunologic reaction involving T-cell pathways. Clinical manifestations are delayed in onset.

8. **B. Piedra is a superficial mycosis of the hair shaft. White piedra is caused by *Trichosporon beigelii.*** Black piedra is caused by *Piedraia hortae.* Pityriasis versicolor is a superficial fungal infection of skin caused by *Malassezia furfur.* Tinea nigra is a superficial infection of the epidermis caused by *Phaeoannellomyces werneckii* (*Exophiala werneckii*).

9. **D. Chancroid is a sexually transmitted disease caused by *Haemophilus ducreyi.*** Scraping the base of an ulcer, Gram staining the scrapings, and examining under a microscope will reveal gram-negative coccobacilli singly or in "schools of fish." *Phaeoannellomyces werneckii* is the cause of tinea nigra; warts are caused by papillomavirus. Molluscum contagiosum is caused by a poxvirus. Herpes simplex is caused by a herpesvirus.

10. **C. *Pediculus humanus corporis* is the body louse.** *Pthirus pubis* is the pubic louse. *Pediculus humanus capitis* is the head louse. Rarely, lice can transmit epidemic typhus (*Rickettsia prowazekii*), trench fever (*Rickettsia quintana*), and relapsing fever (*Borrelia recurrentis*).

11. **B. Scabies is caused by tiny mites that burrow into skin and lay eggs.** An infection with yellow crusting of skin is suggestive of impetigo. The chickenpox virus can remain dormant within the trigeminal nerve root ganglion and become activated to cause shingles (varicella zoster). Neither fleas nor ticks cause scabies.

12. E. **Erythema infectiosum is caused by parvovirus B19.** Varicella zoster virus causes herpes zoster (shingles). Molluscum contagiosum is caused by a poxvirus. HPVs cause warts.

13. B. Scarlet fever is caused by circulating toxin produced by group A *Streptococcus*. Pastia's lines may be present. There is a diffuse maculopapular rash on the trunk and extremities with flushed cheeks and circumoral pallor. **The disease usually occurs in children, and is characterized by sore throat and fever, followed by enlarged, red tonsils, lymphadenopathy, and white-coated tongue with red protruding papillae ("white-strawberry" tongue).**

14. A. **Syphilis is often called "the great imitator" because the rash can take so many forms.** The primary lesion is a painless chancre, followed a couple of months later by a secondary stage, a nonpruritic rash that covers the trunk and extremities. Syphilis is caused by *Treponema pallidum*, a spirochete. Syphilis is often associated with alopecia with a "moth-eaten" appearance. Cases of syphilis must be reported to the local health department, where treatment and follow-up of contacts is conducted.

15. C. **Rocky Mountain spotted fever is a dangerous infection that must be recognized and treated.** It is caused by *Rickettsia rickettsii*, which is transmitted by tick bite. Fever and chills occur first, followed about 4 days later with an erythematous, maculopapular rash. In contrast to most infectious rashes that usually begin on the neck and trunk and spread peripherally, the rash of Rocky Mountain spotted fever begins around wrists, hands, and ankles and spreads centrally to the trunk and extremities. There may be petechiae and ecchymoses. Treatment is with tetracycline, tetracycline analogues, or chloramphenicol. Treatment decisions should be made based on clinical and epidemiologic clues and should not be delayed while waiting for confirmation of laboratory results.

16. E. **All of the above. Kawasaki's disease is an acute, vascular disease of unknown etiology that occurs during childhood.** "Cherry red lips" and "strawberry tongue" are characteristic of this disease. Fever is followed by a morbilliform eruption. There may be an erythematous, desquamating rash on the perineum. There is often edema and erythema of hands and feet. Myocarditis, pericardial effusion, and coronary artery aneurysms can occur. Conjunctival injection is usually present. Diagnosis is by clinical presentation.

17. D. Atopic dermatitis is a chronic disorder that usually begins in childhood. It is is often associated with a family history of atopic dermatitis. It is extremely pruritic. In babies, lesions of

atopic dermatitis are often found on the lateral aspects of arms and on cheeks. As the child becomes old enough to scratch, lesions are found in the antecubital fossae, on the abdomen, and in the posterior fossae. **Superimposed infection with *Staphylococcus* or *Streptococcus* often occurs.**

18. E. **Toxic epidermal necrolysis is at the severe end of the spectrum of hypersensitivity reactions.** Nikolsky's sign is present wherein blisters spread with pressure, indicating easy separation of the epidermis from underlying dermis. The body reacts severely, shedding the entire epidermis of skin in sheets, causing fluid loss and severe risk for superimposed bacterial infection. The mortality rate is high. Treatment is that of a burn patient; the patient should be placed in the burn unit of the hospital.

19. D. Pruritic urticarial papules of pregnancy is a hypersensitivity reaction during pregnancy characterized by a pruritic eruption of erythematous and edematous papules that typically develops during the third trimester of pregnancy. **The rash will usually resolve after delivery of the baby.**

20. B. **Herpes gestationis is characterized by annular or serpentiginous lesions composed of bullae or vesicles that extend over the abdomen, to other parts of the trunk, and to extremities.** Herpes gestationis is not caused by the herpes virus. It is an autoimmune disease that occurs during pregnancy or immediately following pregnancy. It is extremely pruritic. Presence of this disorder does not appear to pose significant risk to the fetus.

21. 1E, 2D, 3A, 4G, 5F, 6C, 7B

22. 1B, 2D, 3A, 4C

23. 1F, 2C, 3G, 4A, 5B, 6D, 7E

24. 1H, 2C, 3F, 4A, 5D, 6B, 7G, 8E

25. 1C, 2F, 3E, 4A, 5H, 6B, 7G, 8D

Topical Medications Commonly Used in Dermatology

Topical Corticosteroids

Application of topical corticosteroids is usually twice a day. There are seven classes of potency, with class 1 strongest and class 7 most mild. Within each class, the potency of the steroids are generally the same. Ointments penetrate skin more effectively than creams and are useful on dry areas, but creams are often more cosmetically appealing (less greasy). Class 1 steroids should not be used for more than 2 weeks at a time because of risk for skin atrophy and striae. After discontinuation of class 1 steroids for 2 weeks (during which time a less potent steroid can be applied), class 1 steroids can be reapplied if necessary for another 2-week period. Only class 6 and 7 steroids should be used on the face, in the groin, and in the axilla because of potential skin atrophy on face and increased skin and systemic absorption in the axilla and groin.

■ Class 1 (most potent)

Betamethasone dipropionate (Diprolene) 0.05% cream or ointment
Clobetasone propionate (Temovate) 0.05% cream or ointment
Diflorasone diacetate ointment (Psorcon) 0.05%

■ Class 2 (potent)

Desoximetasone (Topicort) 0.25% cream, gel, or ointment
Fluocinonide (Lidex) 0.05% cream, gel, or ointment
Mometasone furoate (Elocon) 0.1% ointment

■ Class 3 (potent)

Amcinonide (Cyclocort) 0.1% cream and lotion
Betamethasone valerate (Valisone) 0.1% ointment
Fluticasone propionate (Cutivate) 0.005% ointment
Halocinonide (Halog) ointment 0.1%
Triamcinolone acetonide (Aristocort A) 0.1% ointment

■ **Class 4 (mid-strength)**

Flurandrenolide (Cordran) 0.05% ointment
Fluocinolone acetonide (Synalar) 0.025% ointment
Hydrocortisone valerate (Westcort) 0.2% ointment
Mometasone furoate (Elocon) 0.1% cream
Triamcinolone acetonide (Kenalog) 0.1% cream

■ **Class 5 (mid-strength)**

Betamethasone valerate (Valisone) cream 0.1%
Flurandrenolide (Cordran) 0.05% cream
Fluocinolone acetonide (Synalar) cream 0.025%
Fluticasone propionate (Cutivate) 0.05% cream
Hydrocortisone butyrate (Locoid) cream 0.1%
Hydrocortisone valerate (Westcort) cream 0.2%
Triamcinolone acetonide (Kenalog) lotion 0.1%

■ **Class 6 (mild)**

Alclometasone dipropionate (Aclovate) 0.05% cream or
ointment
Desonide (Desowen) cream 0.05%
Desonide (Tridesilon) cream 0.05%

■ **Class 7 (mildest)**

Dexamethasone (Decadron phosphate) 0.1% cream
Hydrocortisone (Hytone) 0.5%, 1.0%, 2.5% cream
Methylprednisolone (Medrol) 1%

Topical Antiseptic and Antibacterial Agents

■ **Antiseptics**

Antiseptics reduce numbers and activity of bacteria and are useful for hand scrubs and skin scrubs for procedures.

- Ethyl and isopropyl alcohols: reduce surface microorganisms; short duration of action.
- Chlorhexidine (Hibiclens): active against gram-positive and gramnegative bacteria as well as some fungi and yeast; long acting.
- Iodine compounds (Betadine): effective against bacteria, fungi, viruses, protozoa, and yeast; long acting; may lose effectiveness upon contact with blood; use in neonates should be avoided.
- Hexachlorophene (Phisohex): bacteriostatic effective against gram-positive organisms; long acting; should not be used on infants or excessively by pregnant women.

■ **Antibacterial Agents**

- Bacitracin: Interferes with cell wall growth; effective against many gram-positive organisms, but inactive against most gram-negative organisms. Useful for wound care after surgery. Apply two or three times a day.

- Mupriocin (Bactroban) ointment: Active against gram-positive bacteria and some gram-negative bacteria. Efficacious in treating impetigo. Apply two or three times a day.
- Silver sulfadiazine (Silvadene): Bactericidal, useful in treatment of burns.

Topical Antifungals

- Ketoconazole (Nizoral) cream: Fungistatic; effective against a broad spectrum of pathogenic fungi and yeast. Helpful for tinea corporis (body), tinea cruris (groin), tinea pedis (feet), intertrigo (under breast, between buttocks), and other fungal and yeast infections. Apply twice a day.
- Naftifine (Naftin) cream: Active against fungi, less active against yeasts. Has some antiinflammatory properties. Apply twice a day.
- Oxiconazole (Oxistat) cream or lotion: Broad spectrum of activity; activity against some strains of yeast. Apply twice a day.
- Terbinafine (Lamisil) cream: fungicidal. Apply twice a day.
- Thymol solution: bactericidal and fungicidal. Use 4% thymol in absolute ethanol for treatment of *Pseudomonas* infection of nails (greenish discoloration of nails). Apply twice a day.
- Clotrimazole (Lotrimin, Mycelex): Treatment of superficial fungal and yeast infections. Lotrimin can be obtained over the counter. Apply twice a day.

Medicated Shampoos

- Medicated shampoos should be left on 5 to 10 minutes before rinsing.
  - Ketoconazole shampoo
  - Selenium sulfide (Sebulex) shampoo
  - Zinc pyrithione (Zincon, Head and Shoulders) shampoo
  - Capex shampoo
  - Selsun shampoo
- Tar shampoos can be helpful for scalp psoriasis.
  - DHS tar shampoo (0.5% tar)
  - Ionil T Plus (2% tar)
  - Neutrogena T-gel (2%)
  - Pentrax (8.75%)
  - Tegrin (5%)
  - Denorex (9%)

Topical Treatment of Axillary, Palmar, or Plantar Hyperhidrosis

Aluminum chloride hexahydrate (20%) in absolute alcohol (Drysol): apply to dry axilla, palms, or soles at night for 5 nights.

Antipruritic Agents

- Avoid topical antihistamines. These can sensitize the skin and result in hypersensitivity reactions.
- Cetaphil lotion with 2% menthol (compounded) is a soothing antipruritic lotion.
- Sarna lotion (contains camphor menthol) is a commercially available, over-the-counter antipruritic lotion. Use as frequently as necessary.
- Pramoxine and hydrocortisone (Pramosone) 0.5%, 1.0%, or 2.5% foam, cream, aerosol, gel, or lotion can be helpful.

Keratolytic Agents

- Salicylic acid: for treatment of warts, 5% to 20% solution (Duofilm, Occlusal) or 40% salicylic acid plasters (Mediplast)
- Urea: for softening stratum corneum such as in treatment of keratosis pilaris of upper arms or hyperkeratosis of hands and feet, Carmol 10 (15% urea) lotion, ammonium lactate (Lac-Hydrin) cream

Acne Medications

A topical antibiotic is often prescribed along with a benzoyl peroxide (antibacterial) or comedolytic/keratinization-altering (tretinoin) agent.
- Topical antibiotics
  - Erythromycin 2% solution or ointment
  - Clindamycin phosphate 1% (Cleocin T) solution, gel, or lotion
  - Sulfur 5% and sodium sulfacetamide 10% (Sulfacet-R, Novacet lotion)
- Benzoyl peroxide preparations
  - Benzoyl peroxide 5% or 10% (Benzac AC, Desquam E, Pan Oxyl, Oxy5 and Oxy10) wash or gel
- Comedolytic and keratinization-altering agents
  - Tretinoin (Retin-A micro 0.01% cream, Retin-A 0.05% liquid or cream, 0.1% cream, 0.01% gel, 0.025% gel)
  - Azelaic acid 20% (Azelex) cream or gel (Azelex also has antibacterial properties)
- Benzamycin combines 3% erythromycin and 5% benzoyl peroxide. Apply once or twice a day.
- Benza Clin combines 1% clindamycin and 5% benzoyl peroxide. Apply once or twice a day.

D Staging of Melanomas

- Staging determines extent of melanoma.
- Determined by thickness, depth into skin, and spread.
- Thickness of tumor important in predicting prognosis.
- Different staging mechanisms.

Clark Level

Level I: all tumor cells above basement membrane (*in situ*)
Level II: tumor extends to papillary dermis
Level III: tumor extends to interface between papillary and reticular dermis
Level IV: tumor extends between bundles of collagen of reticular dermis
Level V: tumor invasion of subcutaneous tissue (87% metastases)

Breslow Thickness

Thin: <0.75 mm depth of invasion
Intermediate: 0.76 to 3.99 mm depth of invasion
Thick: >4 mm depth of invasion

American Joint Committee on Cancer Staging System for Melanoma (AJCC)

- Based on thickness of tumor (T), extent of spread to lymph nodes (N), extent to which it has metastasized to other parts of the body (M)
- Survival rate, after treatment, for 5 and 10 years, respectively, in italics

Stage 0: melanoma *in situ* (Clark level I): melanoma in epidermis, no spread
Stage IA: localized melanoma ≤1.0 mm, no ulceration (T1a N0 M0) *(95%, 88%)*
Stage IB: localized melanoma (≤1.0 mm, ulceration (T1b N0 M0) *(91%, 83%)* or 1.01 to 2.00 mm, no ulceration (T2a N0 M0) *(89%, 79%)*
Stage IIA: localized melanoma 1.01 to 2.00 mm, ulceration

(T2b N0 M0) *(77%,64%)* or 2.01 to 4.00 mm, no ulceration (T3a N0 M0) *(79%, 64%)*

Stage IIB: localized melanoma 2.01 to 4.0 mm, ulceration (T3b N0 M0) *(63%, 51%)* or >4.0 mm, no ulceration *(67%, 54%)*

The following involve spread of melanoma, any thickness:

Stage IIC: localized melanoma >4.0 mm, ulceration (T4b N0 M0) *(45%, 32%)*

Stage IIIA: 1 node with microscopic involvement, no ulceration (T1a–4a N1a M0) *(70%, 63%)* or 2 to 3 nodes with microscopic involvement, no ulceration (T1a–4a N2a M0) *(63%, 57%)*

Stage IIIB: 1 node with microscopic involvement, ulceration (T1b–4b N1a M0) *(52%, 38%)* or 2 to 3 nodes with microscopic involvement, ulceration (T1b–4b N2a M0) *(50%, 36%)*, or 1 node with macroscopic involvement, no ulceration (T1a–4a N1b M0) *(59%, 48%)*, or 2 to 3 nodes with macroscopic involvement, no ulceration (T1a–4a N2b M0) *(46%, 39%)*, or in-transit metastases/satellites without metastatic nodes, ulceration or not (any T N2c[7] M0) *(47%, 37%)*

Stage IIIC: 1 node with macroscopic involvement, ulceration (T1b–4b N1b M0) *(29%, 24%)* or 2 to 3 nodes with macroscopic involvement, ulceration (T1b–4b N2b M0) *(24%, 15%)* or ≥4 metastatic or matted nodes, or in-transit metastases/satellites and metastatic nodes, ulceration or not (any T N3 M0) *(27%, 18%)*

Stage IV: Metastasis to other parts of the body: (any T, any N, any M, any ulceration) *(<5%)*

Distant skin, subcutaneous or nodal metastases (M1a)

Lung metastases (M1b)

All other visceral or distant metastases (M1c)

View the National Comprehensive Cancer Network (NCCN) guidelines for management of melanoma at www.nccn.org

Index

Note: Page numbers followed by *f* refer to figures; those followed by *t* refer to tables; those followed by *b* refer to boxes.